Personality Dynamics

Personality Dynamics

Benjamin B. Wolman

New York, New York

PLENUM PRESS ● NEW YORK AND LONDON

Library of Congress Cataloging-in-Publication Data

Wolman, Benjamin B.
    Personality dynamics / Benjamin B. Wolman.
        p.   cm.
    Includes bibliographical references and index.
    ISBN 0-306-43956-5
    1. Personality. 2. Developmental psychology. 3. Social
psychology.   I. Title.
BF698.W63   1992
    155.2--dc20   91-38074
                                                         CIP

ISBN 0-306-43956-5

© 1992 Plenum Press, New York
A Division of Plenum Publishing Corporation
233 Spring Street, New York, N.Y. 10013

Printed in the United States of America

Preface

Personality Dynamics endeavors to describe the nature of human nature. My greatest debt is to Sigmund Freud, although my own research and thinking have led me to form fresh hypotheses not always in agreement with Freud's master plan. I do believe that I am following Freud's spirit, although I have introduced a new conceptual system. Freud learned from and rebelled against many theories and ideas of his time; isn't the moral obligation of his disciples to forge ahead and not to follow in his footsteps? Based on new empirical data and scientific discoveries unknown in Freud's time, I have endeavored to develop a new set of concepts and new interpretations of the nature of human nature.

In my over forty years of research, teaching, and practice I had come to realize that no one has the monopoly on truth. I am indebted not only to Freud and Heinz Hartmann but also to those who rejected Freud's system—among them Alfred Adler and Harry Stack Sullivan—and to scores of colleagues, students, and patients who enabled me to look for and discover hitherto unknown aspects of human nature.

The present volume introduces, among other ideas, (1) a new approach to theory formation in psychology; (2) a modified nature–nurture hypothesis in behavior genetics; (3) the principle of monistic transitionism as a possible solution to the mind–body dichotomy; (4) the idea of protoconsciousness; (5) the concepts of Eros and Ares as chief motives in love, hate, and sex; (6) the power and acceptance theory of human relations; (7) the social patterns of instrumentalism, mutuality, and vectorialism; (8) the concept of interindividual cathexis; (9) some ideas concerning mental health and mental disorder; (10) the five stages of moral development: anomy, phobonomy, heteronomy, socionomy, and autonomy; and (11) personality integration concept.

The main aim of this book is to encourage empirical research that will lead to the development of new theoretical constructs in psychological theory and especially in personality dynamics.

I am profoundly indebted to Dr. Joseph Notterman for his constructive criticism and to the editorial staff of Plenum for their efficient cooperation.

BENJAMIN B. WOLMAN

Contents

1

The Logic of Science and Psychological Theory

THE NEED FOR A THEORY

The need for a theory is neither self-evident nor ever-present. One may know a lot of things and never try to go beyond them. One does not need any theory at all in order to call friends, relatives, or business associates, for the telephone book offers the necessary information concerning telephone numbers without forming theories beyond the empirical data described in the telephone directory.

The fact remains, however, that the knowledge of empirical data pertaining to objects and bodies and to what happens to them (facts) is not always as adequate as a telephone directory. Consider the production of cars or the building of houses. *Why* does gasoline make a car go? *What* does the steering wheel do to the wheels of the car? *What* does the switch do to electric lights in a house?

Mere descriptive statements, such as "All cars have a gas tank" or "Light bulbs go on at the turn of a switch," are not of much help. Scientific research started when self-evident

1

empirical data failed. The ancient Egyptians watched floods of the Nile; they knew the facts and could *describe* them with great precision. But when the Egyptians needed to regulate irrigation, they had to seek the not-so-evident and not the easily observable connections. They had to reach *beyond* the observable data and seek *explanations*. In addition to the questions of "what" and "how" things happen, they had to know *why* they happened. Prior to Freud, psychopathology was a collection of descriptive data, sort of a pile of bricks. Freud has added several new bricks (empirical data), but he has also developed an overall theory—he built a house (Freud, 1933, 1949, 1950; Pribram and Gill, 1966).

A theory does not contradict empiricism. Newton was certainly an empirical scientist. Had Newton, however, merely observed that apples fall down (an empirical generalization), his role in the history of science would be rather negligible. Newton's greatness lies in his theory. Newton went beyond empirical findings; he asked the question *why* things fall, and the search for an answer led him to the formulations of a series of *theoretical constructs*, such as force, mass, and gravitation. Without these constructs physics would have remained a pedestrian aggregation of observable facts. Analogously, without Freud, psychopathology would have remained a catalog of observable symptoms. Great scientists do not confine themselves to the discovery of new data; they create conceptual tools that help in fresh discoveries (Jeans, 1958).

Some philosophers of science seem to believe that theory must be arrived at by an inductive method and empirical generalizations. This is not necessarily true, for Newton and Einstein did not arrive at their bold theories through empirical generalizations. The history of psychology knows of several other approaches to theory formation (Gilgen, 1970; Hull,

1943; Lewin, 1936; Rychlak, 1984; Wolman, 1984; Wolman and Nagel, 1965).

FORMING HYPOTHESES

A theory as a set of logical statements is neither true nor false in the empirical sense. It *explains* the empirical data and it must do it according to formal logical rules. The three main rules are: inner consistency of the statements (*immanent truth*); the theoretical statements need not contradict empirical data (*transcendent truth*); and *heuristic usefulness*, which means opening new vistas and producing additional knowledge.

Pavlov and Freud did not subscribe to Kant's critical idealism nor to Comte's positivism; their approach was that of empiricism, but they went beyond the observable data.

A similar approach was taken in astronomy and chemistry: Astronomers proved the existence of celestial bodies before they were discovered. A similar development occurred in the history of other sciences, where hitherto nonobservable elements were discovered not always by pure empirical methods, but by logical deductions (Bohm, 1957; Bridgman, 1936; Feigl, 1951; Fiss, 1979; Nagel, 1961; Wolman, 1981; Wolman and Nagel, 1965).

Scientific laws are established by inference. The processes that psychology deals with

> Are in themselves just as unknowable as those dealt with by the other sciences, by chemistry or physics, for example; but it is possible to establish the laws which those processes obey and to follow over long and unbroken stretches their mutual relations and interdependences—in short, to gain what is known as an "understanding" of the sphere of natural phenomena in question. This cannot be effected without forming

fresh hypotheses and creating fresh concepts. (Freud, 1949, p. 36)

And this is exactly how Freud developed his theory (Wolman, 1984).

There are two historical sources of the pseudoempirical approach in modern philosophy—Comte's positivism and Mach's sensationalism. The struggle between empiricism and rationalism in modern philosophy took an unfortunate turn in Kant's critical idealism. Kant wrote, "Though all our knowledge begins with experience it does not follow that it all arises out of experience" (1929, preface). Kant's solution to the empiricism versus rationalism controversy was to substitute laws of the human mind for laws of nature. Time, space, quantity, causation, and so on became a priori forms of perception of the transcendental mind. In a truly anti-Copernican revolution, Kant put the perceiving mind in the center of the universe. "Take away the thinking subject," wrote Kant, "and the corporeal world will vanish" (1929, p. 00).

Two philosophers expanded Kant's philosophy and brought it to its inevitable logical conclusions. According to Kant, the perceived world was a cluster of phenomena. The world as it really was (*Ding-an-sich*) was impenetrable; the world of phenomena was a result of sensory perception determined by the a-priori-set forms of the perceiving mind. Schopenhauer (1923) went one step further; according to him the world was a creation of one's will and idea (*Wille und Darstellung*). Hegel (1841) "objectified" Kant's philosophy and ascribed the laws of dialectic logic to the universe. According to Hegel, the history of nature and man was supposed to follow the rules of a certain logical system that pleased him.

The history of philosophy after Kant is largely dominated by the efforts to prove or disprove or modify Kant's impact. Empirical scientists like Darwin, Spencer, Pavlov, and Freud dismissed Kantian influence. Freud wrote in 1933 in the *New Introductory Lectures*,

> You can hardly avoid coming to the conclusion that our philosophy has preserved essential traits of animistic modes of thought, such as overestimation of the magic of words and the belief that real processes in the external world follow the lines laid down by our thoughts. It is, to be sure, an animism without magical practices. (1933, p. 226)

Comte and Mach supported three distinct solutions to the problems Kant had created. Comte rejected all epistemological considerations. In the *Cours de Philosophie Positive* (1864), Comte divided the history of human thought into the teleological, metaphysical, and positive eras. In the era of positivism, one was not supposed to test the boundaries of human cognition and ask "why" things happen. Science should be purely descriptive and deal with the question "how" things happen. According to Comte, a theory is a set of *empirical generalizations* arrived at by the use of the inductive method.

Another solution to the Kantian dichotomy of the perceiving subject versus the perceived world was offered by Mach, who wrote:

> Nature is composed of sensations as its elements... no inalterable thing exists. The thing is an abstraction, the name of a symbol.... Sensations are not signs of things, but on the contrary, a thing is a thought symbol for a compound sensation of relative fixedness. Properly speaking, the world is not composed of "things" as its elements, but of colors, tones, pressures, spaces, times, in short, what we ordinarily call individual sensations. (1960, p. 482)

Scientific inquiry must proceed from sensory perception through the search for logical connections between them toward description and prediction. A theory must correspond solely to sensory data. "In a complete theory," wrote Mach, "to all details of the phenomena, details of the hypothesis must correspond, and all rules for these hypothetical things must also be directly transferrable to phenomena" (1911, p. 57).

There was a short step from Mach to the logical positivism with its stress on "sensory data" and "objective language." The true world of bodies and events receded into the background. Instead, logical positivism analyzed sensations and actions. The problem of theory formation was reduced to translating the "intersubjective sensory perceptions" into "objective, physicalistic" language. A realistic cognition of the world was substituted by a formal presentation of scientific propositions. Thus "syntax" and the "logical analysis of language" became the main problems of the philosophy of science. Following, in a way, in Kant's footsteps, the logical positivists renounced the principle of transcendent truth.

EPISTEMOLOGICAL REALISM

While radical empiricists, neopositivists, and operationists insisted that theory be merely a superstructure of sensory data, Darwin, Huxley, Sechenov, Pavlov, Freud, Einstein, and other empirical scientists neither accepted the subjective sensory data as the sole basis for science nor suggested reducing theory formation to a catalog of sensory data.

Einstein advocated the idea proposed by Poincaré (1902) that "fundamental concepts and postulates" in science are "free inventions of the human mind." Theoretical interpretation is not a mere generalization or abstraction from facts: "Every attempt at a logical deduction of the basic concepts and postulates of mechanics from elementary experiences is doomed to failure," Einstein wrote in 1934 (p. 15).

THE IMPACT OF THE SOCIOCULTURAL CLIMATE

Scientists do not live in a vacuum, and scientific theories are man-made cognitive systems related to a particular sociocultural background. Consider the cultural–historical scene of the sensualist versus rationalist philosophy.

René Descartes was concerned with the separation of physics from theology. This was a relevant issue in a time of religious wars and the beginnings of scientific inquiry. Whether Descartes was afraid to express his true feelings in religious matters is still a controversial issue, but Descartes's times were certainly not conducive either to an outright rejection of religion or to an uncritical theological interpretation of the universe. One hundred years later, the Encyclopedists interpreted the world without resorting to religious concepts, but 100 years earlier no one could have known what Descartes learned from Harvey on the nature of living organisms.

Descartes had to divide the world into matter ruled by the mechanical laws of physics of his time and mind ruled by the traditional soul. Descartes's dualism of mind and body bears witness to the gulf between science and religion at that time (Descartes, 1931).

When John Locke embarked on a *sensualist theory of the mind*, he had to face some Cartesian problems. *Introspection* was Descartes's method; "Cogito, ergo sum" ("I think, therefore I am") was Descartes's credo. At that time introspection had become the cornerstone of the new empiricism, but Locke was definitely opposed to the "innate ideas," described by Descartes, Spinoza, or any of the "scholastic men," as Locke named them. According to Locke, the human mind at birth was a *tabula rasa* (clean slate). In his criticism of Descartes, however, Locke could not overcome Descartes's rationalism, and Locke's empiricism was more programmatic than factual (Locke, 1894). Furthermore, Locke's system was empirical only insofar as it was opposed to the rationalist tradition of erecting metaphysical structures unrelated to sensory data.

A history of psychology that deals with psychology and only psychology tells an incomplete and truncated story, for psychology has always been interrelated with philosophy, mathematics, and natural sciences. The history of psychology should be viewed in the perspective of the history of civiliza-tion, with special emphasis on the history of philosophy and science. The cultural–historical continuity will appear to the searching eye in an utmost convincing manner, for each par-ticular scientific issue has always been a link in the chain of human thought and a part of the continuum of human thought. Every single research worker lived in a certain epoch, was influenced by its cultural heritage, and inevitably turned to seek answers to the problems posed by his contemporaries or forerunners (Wolman, 1968). History is not an experimental science, but it seems highly improbable that Einstein's relativ-ity theories could have come into being unless stimulated by the problems posed by Maxwell, Mach, Hertz, and many others.

RADICAL REALISM

The business of science is to search for truth and to report the results of the research. Any scientific system, including the one to be reported in the present volume, must make explicit both how it has arrived at the conclusions and how it will go about reporting them.

One must clarify the fundamental tools one has used on the long journey from the inception of research to the reporting of the results. The aims of the journey are the first things that require explanation. As stated above, truth is the sought-after goal; what is, then, the so-called truth?

For centuries, philosophers attacked the problem of truth and offered a variety of solutions. The epistemological assumption underlying the theories developed in the present volume is that *things are what they are* regardless of whether someone does or does not perceive them. In other words, the conviction expressed here is that America existed before Columbus. Columbus did not create America; he merely discovered it. Or, as Einstein (1934) wrote, "The belief in an external world independent of the percipient subject is the foundation of all science."

This position of *radical realism* is far from the naive realism that assumes that things are perceived. Radical realism is aware of the perceptual inadequacies of a certain biological species that is capable of verbalizing its perceptions. This species, *Homo sapiens,* has no monopoly on perception of the world. The hunter perceives the wolf and acts accordingly; the wolf perceives the hunter and also acts accordingly. If wolves could talk, their theory of human behavior could certainly be enlightening, although it would be greatly influenced by their acuity of sensory perception and ability to reason. Human cognitive talents are likewise limited; human perception and reasoning are often fallacious. There is no reason to assume that our senses never err.

Without the assumption that things and events (that is, what happens with things) are independent of the perceiver, any further discussion of scientific procedures would be rendered useless. Scientific research can be defined as action (behavior) leading toward the development of a system of true propositions constituting science or the scientific system. Should one accept Schopenhauer's (1923) epistemological premise that the world is a product of the perceiver's will and imagination, scientific inquiry would become impossible. If the perception of the world as it is, is impossible and what we perceive is only determined by our mind, "objective research" would be a meaningless term.

TYPES OF LOGICAL PROPOSITIONS

Logicians distinguish between analytic and synthetic statements, or propositions. *Analytic* propositions (also called *definitions*) are not related to objects and bodies but to facts, that is, what happens with them. Analytic propositions can be true or false, irrespective of whatever factual information they convey. Consider the following propositions: "If the train has ten cars, and John rides in the last car, then John rides in the tenth car," or "The name of this man is John or not John," "Paris is in France, and if France is a part of Asia, Paris is in Asia," and so on.

Synthetic propositions (also called *descriptive*) are true only if they agree with facts. For instance, "Paris is in Asia" is a false proposition. The last part of the following proposition is true, in all circumstances: "If people are descendants of butterflies, they walk on two legs." The second part of the above sentence is always true, irrespective of the antecedent part.

I have elsewhere (Wolman, 1973, pp. 42–43) described the various types of propositions sciences use as follows:

1. Synthetic propositions describing *directly observable behavior,* such as overt acts of love, violence, learning, and so on.
2. Synthetic propositions describing *introspectively observable behavior,* such as feelings of attachment, planned

genocide, contemplated suicide, and so on. Despite the opposition to Wundt's and Titchener's reliance on introspection, psychology cannot afford to exclude covert behavior from its realm of study.

3. Synthetic propositions describing *inferrable unconscious behavior*, such as hidden displacements of fear, repressed incestuous desires, and so on. Unconscious phenomena are not easily accessible, yet their existence cannot be denied, and empirical sciences deal with all that exists whether it is visible or not.

4. The above-mentioned types of propositions could apply to groups, classes, and categories of behavior, thus becoming synthetic propositions conveying *empirical generalizations*. These generalizations were called "empirical laws" by Feigl (1951) and "experimental laws" by Nagel (1961).

Actually empirical statements are not "laws" but mere inductive generalizations. Consider such statements as "Hereditary traits are carried by genes," "Newborn children can suck," "Most manic-depressives harbor suicidal thoughts," "Dreams apply pictorial symbolism," and so on.

Empirical generalizations can be arrived at by naturalistic observation, measurement, surveys, statistical studies, and experimentation. Empirical generalizations in psychology may not be as simple as they seem to be. Take, for example, the following cases: "Whenever you hit a windowpane with a hammer, you break the glass." Whenever p, then q, or $p \supset q$; p stands for the first proposition, q for the second. Now substitute "iron door" for "windowpane." Apparently "iron" would not break. Thus, whenever p, then not q, or $p \supset q'$ p stands for the proposition, "A hammer hit the iron door," and q' stands for "The iron door did not break."

Now let us substitute a person for the "windowpane." So far as physiology and anatomy are concerned, the issue might be presented as follows: "The skin was bruised, there was some bleeding, swelling, and eventually damage to a bone."

What happens to people when they are hit by someone? Were a man a simple organism, his reaction would be fight or flight. But people react in different ways. One may start a verbal argument, rationalize, negotiate, forgive, plan revenge, blame himself, and take several courses of action. Thus general statements such as "Hurt men cry," "Hurt men blame themselves," are not true if "men" means "all men." It may be true in regard to "some men," but even the same man may react in different ways.

THEORY FORMATION

Theories operate with a fifth category of propositions. Theoretical statements are *analytical*, for they do not convey empirical data. They go beyond them.

A mere description of objects and facts is a rather incomplete knowledge. A mere collection of facts resembles a pile of bricks; it is not a house. A builder uses bricks to build a house; scientists link the facts, integrate them, and build a theoretical system (Poincaré, 1902).

Were it possible to build a scientific system by empirical generalization, there would be no need for theoretical propositions. Unfortunately, such a purely empirical system is impossible. Consider physics: Gravitation, the corpuscular theory of light, the electromagnetic field theory, and the quantum and relativity theories are not empirical generalizations. Stating that all bodies fall with the same speed in a vacuum is an empirical generalization; so is the observation that apples fall but feathers and balloons rise. Empirical generalizations concern observable facts only; they state what happens and how. But science must reach beyond observable data, develop inferences about unobservables, and discover connections and relationships. These inferences and hypotheses enable us to relate present events to past and future events.

Such a procedure is no longer observation or generalization from observation. It involves filling loopholes in observations, bridging gaps by means of experiments, and relating things that are, as far as empirical data are concerned, not related. It is no longer purely empirical research; it is theory formation. Modern astronomy and physics are as much indebted to deductive, theoretical concepts as to inductive, empirical generalizations (Rowan–Robinson, 1981). The discovery of outlying planets in the solar system was brought about by theory.

Einstein's relativity theories and the space-time continuum are not direct products of observation or experimentation. Discussing Bridgman's operationism, Einstein (1959) wrote:

> In order to be able to consider a logical system as physical theory it is not necessary to demand that all of its assertions can be independently interpreted and "tested operationally"; *de facto* this has never yet been achieve by any theory and can not at all be achieved. (vol. 2, p. 679)

A theory is a set of hypothetical propositions that are not derived from empirical data. Empirical data are *statements* of facts; a theory is not a statement of facts but an *explanation* of facts. It is a fact that solid bodies turn into fluids under the impact of heat, but there are tremendous differences as to why ice, copper, and aluminum melt. *The "why" is no longer a matter of fact, but an explanation of fact.*

All sciences use *intervening concepts.* Lewin wrote:

> In physics, e.g., such terms as "force," "energy," "momentum," and "quantity" are names for facts which cannot be directly perceived, but which are properties representing certain types of reaction or behavior. It is fair to say, I think, that there never has been a psychological school which did not make use of such intervening concepts such as "association," "instinct," "libido," "drive," etc. It is an illusion to believe that it is possible to develop on a purely empirical basis any science which deals with questions of interdependence and causation, if one understands by empiricism the exclusion of theories. None of the psychological systems thus far developed has been "empirical" in this sense. Consequently, instead of attempting to follow the mystical ideal of a "purely empirical" science of "facts" without theories or concepts, one may as well face openly and without disturbance the "fact" that dynamic constructs have been unavoidable in any worthwhile psychology. Why not then introduce these concepts in a deliberate and orderly fashion, rather than permit them to slip in secretly and uncontrolled by the back door? (Lewin, 1938, p. 12)

A theory is neither true nor false in an empirical sense. It is a system of hypothetical constructs, models, and definitions. Its data are usually reported in analytic propositions. Hull's "drive" and Pavlov's "coupling," "conditioning," and "irradiation" are hypothetical constructs. Freud's structural theory and its components—id, ego, and superego—is a complex model of personality.

A theory cannot be empirically proved or disproved. It may be arrived at by chance, as happened with the falling apple that inspired Isaac Newton's theory of gravitation. It can be arrived at in an inductive or deductive manner. A treasure is a treasure, no matter how it is found.

There are several criteria for the acceptability of a scientific theory. The first criterion is the principle of *immanent truth*, an outgrowth of the Aristotelian *tertium non datur*. A scientific theory must represent a system of propositions free from inner contradictions.

The second criterion for acceptability of a scientific theory is its relationship to observable data. If someone were to explain migratory trends by the influence of invisible little ghosts, there would be no need to refute such a theory. Therefore, the principle of *transcendent truth* requires that the system of propositions be free from contradiction with data obtained by observation or experimentation.

Whereas the principle of immanent truth is self-evident and generally acceptable, the principle of transcendent truth is one of the most controversial issues in contemporary philosophy of science. Certainly, one can hardly expect, from a contemporary philosopher, the reply Hegel gave to the criticism that his theory was contrary to historical facts and reality. Hegel's famous reply was "Desto schlimmer für die Wirklichkeit" (too bad for reality) (Hegel, 1841).

Yet even the acceptance of the principle of transcendent truth does not solve the problem. The difficulty lies not within the theoretical system but within the empirical data. Some scientists, such as Bridgman (1927, 1936), have insisted that theoretical propositions be checked against data obtained by rigorously controlled experimentation and described in terms of experimental procedures. However, such a demand debars astronomy, geology, paleontology, history, and archaeology from science. Yet, since scientific research activity aims at the discovery of the truth, no part of the universe and no event may be excluded from inquiry.

Moreover, even those sciences that operate with experimental method cannot operate with it exclusively. Thus some aspects of biology are experimental but others are not. It is certainly an unwarranted belief that psychology is an experimental science and nothing else. Certain aspects of human behavior cannot be dealt with by experimental methods; ethical reasons eliminate others from consideration.

In some cases, the efforts to "check" a theory against experimental evidence either have forced the theory into a Procrustean bed of data obtained by a certain experimenter in a certain setting with certain experimental subjects or else have failed to find conclusive evidence in the direction of either proof or disproof. Hull's impressive theoretical system was checked against certain experiments conducted in a certain way with a certain species (rats). On the other hand, experiments conducted by such experimenters as Tolman, Skinner, Razran, Guthrie, and many others could not be used as empirical evidence for Hull's theory. Thus Hull's theory was "proven" only insofar as it has been found in agreement with *certain* empirical data. Its general validity, for both rats and humans, has been questioned by scores of experimental and theoretical workers.

The second type of experimental evidence that has ended up with inconclusive results is the experimental research in psychoanalysis. One cannot but admire the zeal and thoroughness of the studies conducted by several outstanding workers and yet wonder what proof was expected from these studies. Psychoanalytic theory is a system of hypothetical propositions that deal with a few observable facts or symptoms and with a great many inferred and unobservable facts of unconscious life. (Wolman, 1984).

As a set of observational or empirical generalizations, psychoanalysis describes the ambivalence of human nature. People do not necessarily either love or hate; they often practice both at the same time toward the same person. People may try hard to attain a goal and at the same time do everything to thwart their own efforts. People may be domineering and subservient, independent and overdependent, gay and sad at the same time and act in a most illogical way. Freud's theoretical work was certainly not rigorous, but when one deals with "the most obscure and inaccessible region of the mind, [the] least rigid hypothesis...will be best" (Freud, 1949, p. 2).

Psychological theories operate with a complex set of hypothetical constructs and models. For example, the statement that anxiety is a state of tension created by a conflict between the ego and the superego is not an observable fact but a hypothetical construct. Reinforcement, drive, habit, irradiation, and concentration are likewise not empirical facts but hypothetical constructs. Hypothetical constructs cannot be directly validated; there is no shortcut between them and empirical generalizations; special "correspondence rules" must be established. These rules can be formulated in several ways, depending on the nature of the empirical data (Nagel, 1961, pp. 97*ff*).

A theory does not deal directly with observables but with "empirically unobservable, purely imaginative or intellectually known, theoretically designated factors, related in very complicated ways to the purely empirically given" (Northrop, 1959). Psychological theory must find its own, very complicated ways or "correspondence rules" between theoretical constructs and empirical generalizations.

Certain aspects of modern philosophy of sciences developed out of research and concepts of theoretical physics do not apply to psychological data. Every psychological theory must deal independently from physics with the problems of causality, reductionism, driving forces, and field-theory (Eccles, 1953; Filskov and Boll, 1981; Gilgen, 1970;

Irani, 1980; Lewin, 1938; Maslow, 1968; Rychlak, 1984; Wolman, 1981).

CAUSALITY

The causal principle offers a link between empirical data and theory. Causation binds empirical data in temporal sequences, and the causal continuum permits one to present events or actions in such a way that each event can be seen as a total or partial effect of antedating events and, at the same time, as a total or partial cause of future events. In a causal chain, the present events will be explained by an answer to the question "Why did it happen?" The future events are predicted by the answer to the question "What will be the outcome of the present events?" (Bohm, 1957; Nagel, 1961; Popper, 1961; Wolman, 1981).

The doubts regarding the meaning of *temporal sequences* that perplex physics, especially quantum theory and Einstein's concept of time as the fourth dimension, are not related to psychology. Psychology deals with living organisms, and life has its well-defined starting point and a very deadly deadline. The life span of an organism follows the sequences of beginning by hatching or birth, then growth and phasic changes, and ultimately death, either natural or caused by physical, chemical, or other factors. Every life process contains definite *temporal sequences*. The march of life is measurable in lunar or solar years, in a series of clearly distinguishable sequences of "before" and "after."

Thus an empirical–realistic psychologist tries not only to describe but also to explain hostile behavior, overt and covert alike. He may relate it to a general principle of *constancy* as Freud did, or he may seek organic roots of hostile impulses as Hartmann proposed. This is not to say that he cannot look for other interpretations.

The principle of causation is most likely to offer definite methodological advantages in psychology. It suffices to state here that any theory of motivation, whether Pavlov's, Hull's, or Freud's, is inescapably coined in terms of the causal principle and thereby links present empirical data to past and future data in a necessary and temporal sequence. Pavlov, Freud, Hull, Piaget, and many other productive research workers in psychology have proven by their works the usefulness of the deterministic approach to the study of psychological data.

A dualistic approach would render any psychological inquiry impossible. There are, however, several proposals to bridge over the mind–body gulf and a great variety of reductionistic systems. Despite all the theoretical differences, neither Freud nor Pavlov nor any other serious student of human life could dismiss the fact that all life processes represent a continuum of mind and body.

Freud's personality model fits well into a monistic theoretical framework (Pribram and Gill, 1966; Wolman, 1984). Living organisms can be seen as reservoirs of physicochemical and mental energies. It is assumed that mental energy, phylogenetically, is a derivative of physical energy. In higher organisms there is a continuous *transition* (Freud referred to it as a "mysterious leap") from physical to mental and vice versa (Irani, 1980; Pribram and Gill, 1966; Wolman, 1988).

DRIVE

Let us call the mechanism that activates the discharge of mental energy, drive (or instinctual drive). A theory of drives must fit into a general theory of behavior (principle of immanent truth) and must explain well-established empirical data (principle of transcendent truth), while at the same time being methodologically useful.

A theory of drives must be related to several psychological issues, such as the issue of (1) innate, unconditioned, unlearned reflexes, (2) conditioned reflexes, and (3) cathexis of mental energy. All behavior is a combination of inherited, behavioral tendencies and conditioning. But even these two factors do not explain the totality of behavior.

The term "heredity" includes several separate elements. The first group of factors is the physicochemical constitution. This constitution, however, is not an inflexible entity. It undergoes profound changes in one's lifetime. Every living organism undergoes the process of growth and maturation. This process is typical for each species. In insects it is egg, larva, cocoon, adult insect. In mammals it is conception, intrauterine life, birth, childhood, adulthood, old age, death. In human beings these stages are more distinct, more involved and subdivided.

THE PSYCHOSOCIAL FIELD

Human behavior does not take place in a vacuum. From birth to death human beings interact with other human beings and hardly if ever can human behavior be interpreted in total isolation from social interaction. Even the most objective experimental and clinical studies cannot overlook the impact of the observer on the observed. Whether the researcher calls his observations "participant" or "nonparticipant," the fact of his physical presence affects the behavior of the observed.

Consider the difference in data reported by Freud and Sullivan. Both were keen observers; however, not only their interpretations but even their mere descriptions of the behavior of mental patients were not the same.

The reclining position of the neurotic patient and the sparse communication from the most silent psychoanalyst facilitated transference phenomena. Freud, the keen observer, noticed them and made them the cornerstone of his therapeutic method. However, when a psychotic patient was asked to recline with a psychoanalyst sitting behind his couch and watching him, a different reaction took place. Silence was probably perceived as rejection, and the invisible analyst became a threatening figure. The patient withdrew even more into his shell, and if he did communicate, he would not dare to communicate his true feelings. Such a behavior gave the impression of narcissistic withdrawal and lack of transference feelings toward the psychoanalyst.

Sullivan worked in a hospital where patients were moving back and forth and were acting out their feelings. He saw his patients in interpersonal relations, and being a keen observer, he did not fail to notice the socially induced changes in their behavior. The here-and-now interaction became the clue to the understanding of the patient. Most probably what has been observed in participant observations was not the patient as an isolated entity but the patient in interaction with the therapist, in a *psychosocial field* situation (Wolman, 1967).

Even a nonparticipant observation cannot escape the field situation. Caudill (1958), Stanton and Schwartz (1951), and others conducted extensive nonparticipant observations in mental hospitals. The observers did not treat the patients they observed, nor did they directly participate in making decisions in regard to the observed patients. Yet their very presence influenced, to some extent, the patients' actions.

Needless to say, this influence grows when the interaction is direct and intense. Several research workers have noticed that mental patients, especially schizophrenics, are highly sensitive as to who administers a test and how. Garmezy (1952), Winder (1960), Bellak and Fielding (1978), Wolman (1985), and many others have noticed that the performance of schizophrenics largely depends on who tests them and how it is done and on who interviews or interacts with them (Wolman, 1966). In other words, schizophrenic performance has its ups and downs, depending on rapport. This should not be surprising; Pavlov's dogs became conditioned not only to the metronome but also to the footsteps and to the presence of Pavlov's coworkers. It should be expected that human reactions depend on who the person interacts with and on the emotional tone of such an interaction.

Interaction includes the totality of social experiences of an individual in his lifetime. Whether one stresses or minimizes the importance of hereditary factors, the fact remains that humans do not live in a vacuum and that they interact with others all their lives.

The striking differences in performance between patients who have been recently admitted to a hospital and the long-time "chronic" patients illustrate this. Some students of this issue go as far as to hypothesize that the grave deterioration is a result of hospitalization. Noyes and Kolb (1959) remarked of the chronic schizophrenic patients in the back wards of mental hospitals that their "deterioration is, to a considerable degree, often a hospital artifact" (p. 419).

In physics, under Einstein's influence, there has been a growing awareness of the fact that any observer–observed situation represents a field. Jeans wrote:

> Every observation involves a passage of a complete quantum from the observed object to the observing subject, and a complete quantum constitutes a not negligible coupling between the observer and the observed. We can

no longer make a sharp division between the two....
Complete objectivity can only be regained by treating
observer and observed as parts of a single system. (1958,
p. 143)

Chapters 2, 3, and 4 of this book will further develop and
apply the above-mentioned hypothetical or theoretical constructs (I use these two terms interchangeably) in an effort to
develop a psychological theory that would meet the criteria
of immanent truth, transcendent truth, and heuristic value.
Thus emphasis will be put on building adequate "correspondence rules" that will link the constructs and models to
observable data and, whenever necessary, introduce new hypothetical constructs.

2

Monistic Transitionism

CHANGE AND CONTINUITY

It would be an oversimplification to assume that all aspects of human behavior can be reduced to a simple factor. There is no reason to believe that lack of satisfaction in one direction can be compensated by satisfaction in another, or that mental energy blocked in one direction can be readily transferred to another.

Human behavior is related to the most complex nervous tissues and it depends on a great many biochemical and biosocial factors. Psychologists study living organisms from a certain angle, and recognize that there are *several different* factors that cannot be reduced to one common denominator. There are several valid reasons to be explained later in this book that militate against reducing human behavior to a single factor, or to a single theoretical viewpoint. Human behavior should be viewed in a perspective of evolutionary development that covers a great many diverse factors that could be, probably, presented as follows: (1) At a certain point of evolution the inanimate, nonorganic matter undergoes changes and becomes (2) organic, as described in experimen-

25

tal studies of Oparin (1957). Then, at a certain phase of evolution, matter turns into (3) psychological processes that can be called behavioral.

Human behavior can go either way: from body to mind or from mind to body. For example, human feelings change under the impact of alcohol, and under the impact of human feelings, body chemistry may change. Nature crosses the bridge from mind to body and from body to mind every day in a series of psychosomatic and somatopsychic phenomena (Wolman, 1988).

These principles, which I have called "monistic transitionism," can be summarized as follows:

1. The change does not disrupt continuity of the universe.
2. The unity of the universe remains always the same in a continuous process of change.
3. Biological evolution is a particular case of the universal process of change that may go in any direction, from energy to matter, from mind to body, from past to future, and vice versa.
4. Mind and body are two levels of transition, the mind being a higher level of evolution.
5. Higher evolutionary levels incorporate the lower ones but not vice versa. Thus both theoretical and methodological reductionism must be limited to clearly reducible issues.

Soviet experiments in interoceptive conditioning (Bykov, 1957) prove that the viscera are closer to the unconscious than to the conscious. The inner organs can be conditioned without the subject being aware of it. For example, in an experiment performed by Balakshina (Bykov, 1957) denervated kidneys with a destroyed hypophysis, the physiological processes in kidneys could be interpreted in terms of physics. In experiments on pain reception, where speech signals were used, the role of the cerebral cortex was established. Stimulation of exteroceptors has usually been accompanied by a "subjectively perceived sensation." In Russian psychology, this term denotes mental processes. Stimulation of interoceptors is either not perceived subjectively at all or, at least, not accompanied by any definite, localized perception. Soviet research contributes to the differentiation of what might be called "levels" in the transition from organic to mental. Interoceptive conditioning in man was proven to be unconscious (Bassin, 1968; Chertok, 1981; Razran, 1957; Ziferstein, 1983).

John Eccles, in *The Neurophysiological Basis of Mind* (1953), introduced the hypothesis of the mode of operation of "will" on the cerebral cortex:

> A great part of the skilled activity evolving from the cerebral cortex is stereotyped and automatic, and may be likened to the control of breathing by respiratory centers. But it is contended that it is possible voluntarily to assume control of such actions. (p. 000)

Eccles proposed a theory of how a minute "will-influence," affecting "a single neuron" in the cortex, would trigger off very considerable changes in brain activity. The trigger action can affect neurons which are "critically poised" in unstable equilibrium, just below the threshold of discharging a nerve impulse. In view of the fact that there are some 4,000 neurons packed together per square millimeter (approximately 1/700th of a square inch) of the cerebral cortex and that each neuron has several hundred synaptic connections with other neurons, we have a network of such density and complexity that in the active cerebral cortex the pattern of discharge of even hundreds of thousands of neurons would be modified within 20 milliseconds as a result of an "influence" that initially caused the discharge of merely one neuron. This fact supports the hypothesis that the "will" modifies the spatiotemporal fields of influence that become affected through this unique detector function of the active cerebral cortex.

Eccles quoted the experiments of Rhine, Thouless, Soal, and others as evidence for a generalized "two-way traffic" between mind and matter and for a direct traffic between mind and mind. Eccles believes that extrasensory perception and psychokinesis are manifestations of the principle that allows an individual to influence his own brain, and the brain to give rise to conscious experiences.

SLEEP AND DREAMS

Dreams are one of the main areas where mind and body phenomena cross the dividing line and prove that there is but one universe of interaction and transition. The discovery of rapid eye movement (REM) sleep in 1933 was a milestone in dream research. It has proven beyond doubt that sleep protects dreams and not vice versa. Dream researchers have discovered the cyclical nature of sleep and the role of two organic states, the REM and the non-REM stages. Heart rate, blood pressure, and respiration are irregular and somewhat elevated in REM sleep. Cortical blood flow, brain temperature, and oxygen consumption are lower in non-REM sleep; the twitches of small facial and limbs muscles as well as penile erection are absent in non-REM sleep. The *nuclei raphe* nerve cells in the brain stem control the non-REM sleep. The *locus coeruleus* nerve cells in the brain stem control the REM sleep. The neuron firing in the visual part of the cortex is the same in REM sleep and in the waking state, and is lower in non-REM sleep.

The discovery of lucid dreams (LaBerge, 1984) has opened new vistas in dream research and personality theory. The dichotomy between sleep and wakefulness has been challenged by research on lucid dreams. Lucid dreamers are asleep; they are definitely not awake and therefore they cannot be conscious. They are, however, aware that they are dreaming and therefore they cannot be unconscious. Moreover, lucid dreamers are capable of volitional acting, of clear reasoning, and adequate memory. Obviously they are not unconscious.

The psychoanalytic theory of personality stresses three fundamental determinants—dynamics, topography, and structure. Dynamics deals with the driving forces and the energies they use. *Eros* and *Thanatos* are the driving forces and *libido* and *destrudo* represent the energies at their disposal. Freud's topographic theory deals with the "mental layers" of conscious, preconscious, and unconscious. The structural theory introduces the three "mental agencies," namely, the id, ego, and superego. I suggest that Freud's topographic system be revised on the following lines.

First, there is hardly any reason for a distinction between the *conscious* and the *preconscious* layers. Conscious is what one is aware of at the present time; preconscious is what one was aware of and what can easily come back. In other words, what is on one's mind right now is conscious; what is in one's mind but not on one's mind at the present moment is preconscious. Apparently, conscious and preconscious are the same stuff, and preconscious is the storage room of the conscious. Both conscious and preconscious are accessible to reality testing; preconscious is the name for the memory link between the present and the past states of consciousness.

Unconscious is totally different from conscious and preconscious; it is what one is totally unaware of. Freud described a great many unconscious phenomena such as dreams, amnesia, errors of everyday life, and symptom formation. Unconscious is not a hypothesis; it is a fact proven by empirical research. Russian experimental studies of interoceptive conditioning deserve special attention because they come from a source not too sympathetic to Freud's theories (Bykov, 1957; Razran, 1957).

One may revise Freud's topographic theory by analyzing phenomena that were either unknown in Freud's times or about which knowledge was inadequate. Sensory deprivation, biofeedback, and autogenic therapy were then unknown. Transcendental meditation, certain imagery processes, and parapsychological phenomena of telepathy and psychokinesis were not yet scrutinized by rigorous scientific research.

It is my conviction that all these phenomena are neither entirely conscious nor entirely unconscious. They are not conscious because there is no reality testing, yet the individual who experiences transcendental meditation or telepathy is aware that he does experience these phenomena. The dichotomy between being awake and conscious on the one hand and being asleep and unconscious on the other does not do full justice to what human beings experience. Psychomotor epileptics who attack innocent bystanders are both aware and unaware of what they are doing; they are neither unconscious somnambulists nor conscious muggers. Their state of mind is somewhere between conscious and unconscious—it is *protoconscious.*

The protoconscious plays an important role in mental disorders. Several years ago I was teaching resident psychiatrists in a postdoctoral program in a hospital attached to a medical school. One of the young psychiatrists I supervised, Dr. Strang, was having a difficult time with Janice, a paranoid schizophrenic patient. In a meeting with the medical director (I did not take part in this meeting), Dr. Strang announced that he was not making any progress with Janice and refused to continue to treat her. Since no other resident agreed to work with Janice, the medical director decided to send her away from our university hospital to a state hospital. The next morning, when Dr. Strang had a day off, the medical director issued the proper direction to the nursing department.

That morning I came to the hospital two hours ahead of my schedule and went straight to the nurses' station. The head nurse greeted me with an expression of distress. "Janice got wild this morning," she said. "She came calmly to the nurses' station and asked for a pill for a headache. Before the nurses had the chance to give her the pill, Janice attacked them, tearing their aprons, scratching their faces, breaking things, and screaming wildly. The nurses called the guards, who put Janice in a straitjacket and locked her up. Now, she is cursing and screaming!"

I asked the guards to bring Janice to my office, untie her, and wait for her outdoors. She stood at the door staring at the floor. She knew that I was Dr. Strang's supervisor. "Hi, Janice," I greeted her, "I am sorry that they locked you up. Dr. Strang is off today. Could you tell me what happened?"

Janice did not answer. She did not look at me. She stood still, staring with a faraway look in her eyes, and clenched her fists.

I started again. "I know you, Janice, as a quiet and friendly person. Somebody must have hurt you. You must feel horrible. Please, talk to me. I will help you. I will do everything I can to help you. I am so sorry, Janice. Please give me a chance."

Janice raised her head and stared at me. I offered her a cigarette. She refused.

I started again. "I won't let them tie your hands. I won't allow them to lock you up in the isolation room. If you don't feel like talking to me, you may go to your room or to the day room, whichever you prefer. But, please, tell me what happened. I will try to help you."

Janice looked at me. She cried. Her lips began to move, and I heard her mutter, "Soldiriver, soldiriver, soldiriver."

I could not understand her. Apparently, she was trying to tell me something. I felt utterly useless, a total failure, unworthy to teach psychiatry. I felt that all the years of graduate and postgraduate training were wasted on me, that I had not learned anything in seven years of supervision and 20 or more years of research, teaching, and clinical experience. Here in front of me stood an unhappy human being calling for help, and I was blind, deaf, and heartless! Decades of training, and I did not know how to help her!

Suddenly, I had a brainstorm. It did not come from my conscious mind. But it did not come from the unconscious either. The idea was crystal clear, self-evident, absolutely sure. "They sold you down the river!" I exclaimed.

Janice sobbed loudly. I did reach her. We spoke the same language. We communicated at the same protoconscious level.

Janice came over and sat down on a chair I offered her near me. She told me, sobbing, what had happened. She was in love with Dr. Strang, but he did not reciprocate, did not feel anything for her. She still had hoped to win him over when the blow came.

She had had a headache this morning and went to the nurses' station asking for a pill. While she waited for the nurses to get the pill, she overheard two nurses speaking. The two were sitting at a desk writing something, and they did not notice her. One of the nurses wrote a note referring Janice to a state hospital. The nurse said that Dr. Strang requested the transfer because Janice was a "pain in the ass," and he could not stand her. The other doctors agreed with him, and no one wanted to work with her.

Janice felt like she had been struck by a thunderbolt. She tore up the transfer slip, hit one nurse, tore up the other nurse's apron, and attacked everyone else for selling her "down the river."

Janice's actions were not completely conscious, nor were they totally unconscious. She knew what she was doing and remembered her actions, but could not control them. She was in a protoconscious state of mind.

So was I. That morning I had felt I had to rush to the hospital, and I went straight to the nurses' station. My words did not come from my conscious or preconscious mind or from the unconscious. I was in a protoconscious state of mind, joining the mind of the schizophrenic girl.

PARAPSYCHOLOGY

Apparently, parapsychological phenomena belong to the "transitionalistic" area of change and continuity together with hypnosis, dreams, empathy, unconscious, cathexis, and a host of other psychosomatic and somatopsychic phenomena (Wolman, 1986). They are the infant and "the same" infant who grew up and became an adult; they are the seed and the tree; the mind and the body. They do not stand alone; modern physics has accepted the dual nature of light, and Firsoff's (1967) theory of the neutrino offers an important sequitur to Einstein's theory of transformation of energy into matter. According to Firsoff:

> The universe as seen by a neutrino eye would wear a very unfamiliar look. Our earth and other planets simply would not be there, or might at best appear as thin patches of mist. The sun and other stars may be dimly

> visible, inasmuch as they emit some neutrinos.... A
> neutrino brain might suspect our existence from certain
> secondary effects, but would find it very difficult to
> prove, as we would elude the neutrino instruments at
> his disposal.
>
> From our earlier analysis of mental entities, it ap-
> pears that they have no definite locus in so-called "phys-
> ical," or better, gravi-electromagnetic space, in which
> respect they resemble a neutrino or, for that matter, a fast
> electron. This already suggests a special kind of mental
> space governed by different laws, which is further cor-
> roborated by the parapsychological experiments made at
> Duke University and elsewhere. (1967, pp. 63–64)

Parapsychological research will probably greatly contrib-
ute to studies of human life, whether they are conducted from
the organic, biochemical, and neurophysiological side or from
the psychological angle. Parapsychology challenges the traditional concepts of time and causation so well entrenched in
organismic and psychogenic theories. Parapsychology introduces new ideas, but any evaluation of parapsychological
theories and data must be at the present time rather tentative
(Chari, 1986).

INTERINDIVIDUAL CATHEXIS

Whatever exists, exists in a certain quantity although no
one knows how to measure the amounts of emotional energy
one possesses. This amount is probably related to overall
physical resources that are somehow transferable into emotional resources.

These emotional energies can be invested (cathected) in
oneself and/or others. One may overinvest (hypercathexis) in
oneself or others or underinvest (hypocathexis) or any combination of the two.

Freud dealt with the person who invests his libido in others. I suggest broadening the concept and studying the cathected person and the *interindividual cathexis*. The concept of interindividual cathexis is merely a theoretical concept and there are no neurological counterparts to it. It may, however, resemble Pavlov's explanation of reflexes. According to Pavlov (1928), an external stimulus is "transformed into a nervous process and transmitted along a circuitous route (from the peripheral endings of the centripetal nerve, along its fibers to the apparatus of the central nervous system, and out along the centrifugal path until, reaching one or another organ, it excites its activity)" (1928, p. 121). Pavlov's description possibly, can be explained in terms of cathexis of physical energy; the external stimulus transmits a part of its energetic load in the peripheral endings of the centripetal nerve, cathects or charges this nerve ending, and through the circuitous route it cathects the nerve center.

One may but speculate about the interindividual cathexis of mental energy, for there is no empirical proof of cathexis of mental energy, nor can one be sure that a cathexis of mental energy follows the same rules as the cathexis of physical energy. The term "interindividual cathexis" is thus introduced as a theoretical construct and not as an empirical fact.

The concept of interindividual cathexis can serve as a bridge between unobservable, inferable, unconscious and some conscious and observable human interaction. When a mother cares for her child, her emotions can be either introspectionally perceived or, in some cases, even unconscious. Her caring behavior, however, is observable. The concept of interindividual cathexis can be applied in this case as follows: The mother's emotional energy (called by Freud libido) is cathected (changed, invested) in the child.

Is the child on the receiving end of the process? Several studies prove the point that something is going on in the child who is receiving maternal love. Freud described the individual who cathects his libido in others but he did not attempt to explain what happens to the one who receives the cathected libido. When a mother loves her child, her libido is cathected in the image of the child; the loving mother "gives love" to her child and some amount of emotional energy, libido, is given away. Freud dealt with the giving mother, but did not study what happened to the receiving child. Does the child "receive" the love that is "given" him? What happens to the child whose mother does not love him? And what happens when the mother demands love from her child?

The sociologically oriented psychoanalyst Karen Horney stressed the *need to be loved*. When a child feels loved and accepted, he experiences the feeling of *safety*. When a child feels rejected, *basic anxiety* develops. Human activities are guided by both pleasure related to satisfaction of basic needs and safety related to human relationships. According to Horney (1939), people would rather renounce pleasure than safety. Instead of promoting Freudian love, sexual or aim-inhibited, Horney introduced the concepts of protection and safety; in place of Freud's active cathexis of libido, that is, the need to give love, she emphasized the need to be loved.

Sullivan went even further in his thinking. His theory is rightly called a theory of interpersonal relations. According to Sullivan (1953), personality can never be isolated from the complexity of interpersonal relations in which the person lives. Sullivan stressed the concept of *empathy*, described by him as a kind of "emotional contagion or communion" between a child and his parental figures. Thus the infant shows a curious relationship or connection with the significant adult, ordinarily the mother. When the feeding mother is upset, the infant may develop feeding difficulty and indigestion.

Numerous studies have corroborated the fact that being rejected or being loved can affect the child's mental and physical well-being. The studies by Spitz, Bowlby, and others offer convincing proof. The experiences during World War II in London (Burlingham and Freud, 1942) and my own experiences during the same time in Palestine and during the Israeli War of Independence have adduced additional evidence. Infants who receive love develop better physically and mentally than do rejected babies.

There cannot be any doubt that human emotions have their own ways of communication independent of spoken language. Music is one of the roads emotions travel. Happy, lively tunes communicate joy, while Chopin's *March Funebre* inspires sadness and grief.

Verbal communication carries a fraction of what people communicate without words. Facial expression and gestures are overt methods of communication, but all people possess some amount of empathic ability, that is, the ability to receive nonverbal and not-apparent emotional cues and signals.

For several years I have supervised young colleagues, psychiatrists, and clinical psychologists. Those who relied solely on the verbal utterances of their patients did not do too well in their therapeutic work.

The concept of interindividual cathexis can be applied also to social interaction and group dynamics. Some individuals relate to others in order to *receive* whatever they need; the others are *instrumental* in the sense that they supply whatever the individual needs; the receiving individual is a taker who *gets* interindividual cathexis from others. The infant–mother relationship is a prototype of such a libido-taking, instrumental relationship.

As the child grows older, he becomes capable of giving and not only taking. The *mutual,* give-and-take relationship provides for a willing exchange of libido cathexes.

COURAGE TO GIVE

It may sound paradoxical but, within certain limits, it is true that the more energy one uses, the more one has at one's disposal for future use. Imagine two identical twin children identically fed and identical in every aspect. Let us order one of them to exercise every day and otherwise lead an active life and confine the other to bed and impose total passivity. After a few months let them undergo physical examination. Undoubtedly, one could find that the passive child did not save any energy, while the active one grew robust and full of energy.

Energy cannot be stored. People who receive the same amount of physicochemical supplies necessary for survival and adequate functioning can use a certain amount of energy at a given time. They need periodic supplies of food and periods of relaxation, rest, and sleep. Within these limits they can use certain amounts of physical and mental energy. The more energy they use, however, the more becomes available to them, as if scratching the surface opens the door to deeper layers and so on.

The human brain is an enormous storage of energy that can be used in several ways. It is a powerful station receiving and sending out millions of messages in verbal and nonverbal codes. Most human beings do not use their entire mental capacity. They may, however, become much more productive if they are properly stimulated. Increased mental activity opens the gates to the dormant resources. When one actively uses his mind, he opens the door to additional resources never used before.

Mental work does not produce new mental resources but makes available the hitherto hidden resources. Lewin described an experiment in which the experimental subjects were asked to make again and again the same pattern of four lines. Pretty soon the subjects exhibited arm fatigue and poor performance. However, "a change to a different pattern of lines, or to making a picture from these lines, sufficed to wipe out the bodily symptoms of fatigue and to bring about reorganization of the activity" (Lewin, 1936, p. 80).

Obviously, the new and more complex activity had made available additional energies. Simple and easy tasks operate with a minimum energy, using the easily accessible superficial layers. A superficial digging gives few results, but the deeper one digs, the more treasures (oil, coal, metals, etc.) become available. Digging does not create treasures but makes them available. Intensive mental work does not increase one's mental potentialities, but enables the use of more of the potentialities already possessed.

Some people believe that passivity saves their lives and protects their physical and mental health. Nothing is farther from the truth than this idea. Life is action and the more active one is, the better the chances for good physical and mental health (Kahana, 1982).

There comes a time when one must curtail activity. Poor physical health or handicap might impose some restraints. Old age may reduce one's agility. It is not true, however, that old age necessarily brings intellectual deterioration, loss of memory, and personality disturbances. Psychological research has disproved the notion of mental decline in old age, for only *some* individuals suffer from diseases of old age, lumped together under the term *senility*. Senility is often associated with hardening of the arteries, loss of sensual acuity, intellectual decline, and emotional disorders; but normal old age, called *senescence*, is free from all these symptoms. A great many gifted people have reached the peak of their intellectual abilities, creative talents, and emotional stability in old age. Winston Churchill became the prime minister of England at the age of 67, and in subsequent years helped save England and humanity from the Nazi barbarians, and, in his seventies, wrote several magnificent historical volumes. Sigmund Freud developed his best ideas after he reached the age of 67; he continued his creative work until the last days of his life, dying at 83. Pablo Picasso, Marie Curie, George Bernard Shaw, Konrad Adenauer, David Ben Gurion, Charles de Gaulle, Golda Meir, and others retained clarity of thought and mental alertness and vigor well into their old age. (Wolman, 1982).

What, then, is true about growing old? The truth is that there is a gradual slowing down of growth from the day of conception until one's last day on earth. The first days after fertilization of the egg by the sperm represent a rapid process of growth and development. This process continues with a gradual deceleration; the older we are, the more slowly we grow. The postnatal changes in an infant occur at a slower rate than those in prenatal life, and increments in physical and mental growth become smaller and smaller. This is the law of *negative acceleration*.

Physical growth reaches its peak in the late teens; intellectual growth continues longer. Not all individuals reach maturity at the same age, and there are considerable differences in both the speed of development and its ultimate results. All pine trees do not grow with equal speed or attain the same height; the same holds true for human beings.

The older one is, the less weight should be attached to chronological age. One expects that an average 15-year-old boy is more advanced intellectually than an average 10-year-old, but one can hardly ascribe intellectual superiority to a 38-year-old compared with a 33-year-old. On the average, intellectual development as measured by intelligence tests comes to an end around the age of 20 or so. Mentally inferior people reach their peak at an earlier age, but mentally superior individuals continue to grow and develop well into maturity and old age.

Several investigators of sexuality in New York have discovered that normal sexual behavior continues well into the seventies and, in some cases, into the eighties and even later. There seems to be a close correlation between the patterns of sexual behavior in youth and adulthood and its continuation in older age. Most people who have had an active sexual life can continue their sexual activities until very old age.

However, an early decline in intensity and frequency of sexual relations in youth or middle age may cause serious sexual deficiency in old age. Some people reduce the frequency and/or intensity of their sexual encounters in their middle years; sometimes they lose interest in their marital partner, or display less initiative in courtship and sexual foreplay. It is rather difficult in old age to revive lost interest and regain sexual virility and passion, but it is not impossible. I once had in treatment a man who renounced sexual relations in his late forties. He came to my office at the age of 68 and, after a while, regained his sexual desires and prowess.

Basically, the physiological changes of age do not prevent continuation of an active sexual life. Very old men may need a little more time to attain an erection, but they can be capable of sustaining a good erection and obtaining full gratification for themselves and their partners. Older women, too, may need more time to obtain a high degree of arousal and lubrication, but they are as capable of enjoying sex and attaining orgasm as they were in their younger years. Continuous sexual interest and regular sexual activity play a highly important role in one's feelings about oneself and prevent psychological aging. People who have an active sexual life in their old age tend to feel and act younger than their less sexually active agemates. (Wolman and Money, 1980).

Abkhasian men and women do not retire at the age of 65. They carry a full workload until the age of 80, and afterward they are allowed a gradual decrease of working hours.

The high correlation between using energy and the ability to have more energy at one's disposal applies to several fields. One of my former patients, presently a well-known theatrical director, was a drifter doing all kinds of odd jobs until he discovered himself in psychotherapy. The lazy drifter turned into a hard-working, enthusiastic, energetic theatrical figure. Not everyone has musical, literary, or other artistic talents, but most people settle for less than they are, instead of developing their potentialities in whatever direction they can, be it manual or nonmanual skills in which their abilities could develop.

How far we will go and how much we can achieve greatly depends on our inner potentialities and on outer possibilities. These are the bricks, the concrete, and the iron bars from which we can build our little or big house.

The concept of interindividual cathexis represents giving one's emotions, giving love, care, and affection. Helping people means giving away something from oneself. A mother who cares for her child enjoys her vectorial attitude. A woman who feeds her child even when she does not have enough food for herself enjoys the act of giving.

Giving enhances one's self-confidence and self-esteem. Self-confidence implies faith in one's ability to satisfy needs, and self-esteem is the joy and pride derived from one's accomplishments. The child who gets milk and love is happy to have his physical and emotional needs satisfied. He feels protected. But the mother who gives milk and love experiences double joy. First, because her beloved child is happy, and second because it was *she* who made him happy and she enjoys the *power* of giving happiness. As a child she herself was *weak* and needed to be taken care of, but presently she is *strong* and can take care of others.

The more she believes in her power, the more power she has, for her self-confidence and self-esteem open the door to her hitherto dormant energies. The more she gives away, the more of her hidden energy becomes available, and she grows and becomes stronger through giving.

Giving enhances one's feeling of power, for giving is a proof of power. Those who do not give, have nothing to give. Those who give, have. Those who are financially rich can give material goods. Those who are emotionally rich can give affection and kindness. Those who are esthetically rich can give works of art.

The greatest power is the power to protect life, to feed and to care and to give happiness. To give oneself is more important than to give anything else.

Some people are afraid to part with whatever they have. They worry about themselves and live lives in cocoons, wrapped up in themselves. They refuse to give themselves as if hoping that mental frugality will increase their power. But the truth is that the less one does, the less one is capable of doing.

What makes people reach out to their hidden resources? What makes a man into a hero? What inspires a composer to write his best symphony? What makes a mother sacrifice her life for her infant?

You cannot get coal, oil, or gold where none exists. You cannot make a tone-deaf child into a musician. No human action can create nonexisting inner potentialities, but it can activate dormant abilities.

What is the name of the key or keys that can open hidden doors? How can one find them?

3

Motivation and Emotions

RELEASERS OF ENERGY

After a long day's work one may feel tired and drowsy. One's energies seem to be used up, and a good, restful sleep is the only thing on one's mind.

Suppose that suddenly this person hears a prowler breaking into his house. The half-asleep house owner instantly becomes alert. He calls the police, and is no longer tired and sleepy. He checks the doors and windows. He is full of energy and his mind works with great speed. He could not now fall asleep although an hour ago he was half asleep. He chats with the police officers, fully alert.

Fear and anger were the keys that unlocked and released additional sources of energy. It seems that energy is stored in several layers. Boredom reduces access to even the superficial layer, whereas motivation cuts deep and activates even the low-lying strata of energy.

In 1943, World War II workers were requested to work better, and cigarettes, which were rare at that time, were offered as reward for greater speed. The workers increased the output considerably while losing some weight. Motivation did not add energy or calories, but accelerated the release of energy.

During World War II and in the Israeli War of Independence, I saw men and women performing superhuman acts of heroism. I came across an eighteen-year-old girl, a freshman in Teachers College, who demanded to be admitted to active combat duty when her boyfriend was killed. "Now, I must fight for two," she said with determination. I spoke to a badly wounded young man who had carried a walkie-talkie to his unit despite his hemorrhaging. I saw a great many men and women who risked their lives (some of them gave their lives) for a cause dear to them. They were highly motivated by their beliefs and ideals, and their actions drew enormous quantities of energy unavailable in usual circumstances.

Apparently, the balance of energies is a precarious one and depends on several factors. One of them is the total amount of energy *within* the organism at a given time. Obviously, no organism can apply all its energies. Such a "total discharge" similar to an explosion of an atom bomb could possibly lead to a radical evaporation of the total amount of potential energy and consequently to a nervous breakdown.

What takes place in the daily processes studied by psychology can be described as follows: Energies are stored at various levels. One may hypothesize that there are several levels or layers of mental energy, some easily accessible and some available only in states of powerful motivation (Brehm and Self, 1989).

The discharge of mental energies seems to depend on (1) amount and level (quantity) of energy, (2) the relationship between it and the inner and outer stimuli, and (3) the given psychosomatic structure. The interrelationship of these three factors determines human behavior. One may feel tired when the energies stored on a certain level are exhausted.

A new stimulus may stir another level of energy, and a tired individual may suddenly feel bursting with energy and ready for action.

One may be "balanced" while exposed to a certain type of stimulation. This balance can be easily disturbed by a change in stimulating factors. Some stimuli can stimulate only a certain level or a certain quality of energy, whereas some others may dig deeper and connect with more powerful layers of energy. Superficial motivation may activate a shallow layer of energy, whereas a stronger motivation may cut deep into the gold mines of human resources. No human being can use his or her entire storage of energy, but appropriate motivation can activate hitherto unused and seemingly unavailable resources. Pain and pleasure are the basic motivating factors that unlock the gold mines of human energy and stimulate action.

PAIN AND PLEASURE

There cannot be any doubt that pain and pleasure are closely related to the most vital functions of the organism and to its survival. Apparently, pain and pleasure are signals of danger and safety, respectively. A toothache, a headache, or a stomachache usually indicate a decay, a wound, or a malfunction of the affected organ. Practically all diseases, traumas, and other damage inflicted on the organism are accompanied by pain. Severe and life-endangering diseases usually produce unbearable pain. When the organism approaches fire or takes in poisonous substances that jeopardize life, pain is usually experienced.

However, a cavity in a tooth and a toothache are not the same. A cavity may cause the feeling of pain, but the cavity and pain are two different things. A skin burn is accompanied

by pain; even if the pain is removed or alleviated by medica-
tion, the burn still exists, indicating the place where the skin
was damaged. Damage and pain do not always go together.

Pleasure feelings usually signal a smooth functioning of
the organism. The intake of food, water, and fresh air elicits
pleasurable feelings. Removal of pain, discomfort, and tension
are experienced as pleasure.

Pain and pleasure are important factors in motivation
of human behavior. Human being seek pleasure-producing
experiences and avoid painful ones. Several scientists have
expressed the opinion that the pleasure–pain continuum is
identical with the satisfaction–deprivation continuum, and
thus synonymous with the terms of human survival.

Two psychoanalysts, Mann and Semrad, wrote, "The
human being is organized on the prototype of a single cell
which also functions on the pleasure–pain principle" (Deutsch,
1959, p. 132).

Our language does not distinguish clearly between satisfaction of needs and feelings of pleasure. Such words as
satisfaction, gratification, and relief serve both purposes. We
say, "The meal was satisfying," "The cold water was gratifying," without making it clear whether it was a satisfaction of
an organic need or a feeling of pleasure. The same applies to
pain. To be hurt means to suffer damage, whether painful or
not, and at the same time to be hurt means to experience pain,
whether a damage was caused to the organism or not.

Not all organic diseases cause pain. Sometimes a mild
and relatively harmless damage to the organism may cause
severe pain; pain may be perceived from nonexistent limbs
after amputation or from a mild and harmless electric shock.
On the other hand, most severe and dangerous diseases such
as cancer may play havoc with an organism without causing
pain until later stages. Carmichael has noticed that "pricking

a guinea pig fetus with a needle so as to bring a drop of blood may not be so effective in eliciting a response as would be a fine hair applied to a corresponding point" (Carmichael, 1954, p. 297). Obviously, certain parts of the body respond to tactile stimuli but do not respond to pain–pleasure stimuli. Hence damage can be caused without eliciting pain.

Bykov wrote: "It has now been definitely proven that some organs (the visceral peritoneum, the surface of the cerebral cortex, and perhaps some parts of the intestine) are devoid of pain sensibility." However, "the absence of pain receptors does not necessarily mean the absence of other interoceptors" (1957, p. 279).

Several cases of interoperception of damage to the organism without pain, communicated by the unconscious, have been reported in the literature (Eissler, 1955). Razran (1957) pointed to the fact that in the simplest, lowest-level conditioning there is no reward or pleasure. The simple classic conditioning based on dominance can be found in invertebrates, decorticated animals, earliest infancy, and visceral organs.

Several experimental studies confirm this view. Consider Tschakhotine's (1938) report on conditioning of paramecia or Guthrie's (1935) studies on conditioning by contiguity with the exclusion of reward. It can be said, therefore, that a great part of human activity is conducted outside the pain–pleasure continuum. I may add that this is the *prehedonic* level of functioning, though a great many human activities are conducted on the hedonic level and motivated by pain and pleasure feelings.

Freud perceived mental life in a pleasure–displeasure continuum. This continuum was related by Freud to increase and decrease (relief) in the amount of excitation. The demand for an immediate relief notwithstanding, possible consequences were called the *pleasure principle,* and the postponement of gratification dictated by self-preservation was called the *reality principle.*

> Freud wrote in 1920, We have decided to relate pleasure and unpleasure to the quantity of excitation that is present in the mind but is not in any way 'bound'; and to relate them in such a manner that unpleasure corresponds to an *increase* in the quantity of excitation and pleasure to a diminution. (1950, p. 2)

At this point, Freud quoted Fechner's hypothesis that reads,

> Every psychophysical movement crossing the threshold of consciousness is attended by pleasure in proportion as, beyond a certain limit, it approximates to complete stability, and is attended by unpleasure in proportion as, beyond a certain limit, it deviates from complete stability. ...If the work of the mental apparatus is directed toward keeping the quantity of excitation low, then anything that is calculated to increase that quantity is bound to be felt as adverse to the functioning of the apparatus, that is, unpleasurable. (Freud, 1950, p. 4)

Obviously, pleasure and reduction of tension are not identical terms. The Fechner–Freud idea of relief of tension was criticized by Goldstein. Goldstein wrote:

> Freud fails to do justice to the positive aspects of life. He fails to recognize that the basic phenomenon of life is an incessant process of coming to terms with the environment; he only sees escape and craving for release. He only knows the lust for release, not the pleasure of tension. (1939, p. 333)

Murphy (1947), obviously influenced by Sherrington, distinguished preparatory appetite versus consummatory functions. Both are pleasure producing. Maslow (1968) also was critical of the tension-relief theory and emphasized the positive striving toward pleasure.

The experiments of Sheffield and Roby (1950) have shown that animals can be conditioned with the nonnutritive taste of saccharin serving as a reward. Probably the pleasant taste of saccharin was the reinforcing agent.

Such experiences as alcoholism, drug addiction, and overeating prove beyond doubt that people can indulge in pleasurable activities even when these activities bring harm to them. Pleasure and pain may become more powerful motives than protection of life. Hyperalgesic individuals may refuse treatment if it causes too much pain.

It can be hypothesized that in phylogenetic evolution the prehedonic stage antecedes the hedonic one. Most probably lower organisms are incapable of pleasure–displeasure sensations, and yet they function and even can learn. No one could ascribe pleasure to plants or to their vital functions of osmosis, assimilation of carbon, and tropisms.

A great many functions of higher mammals are associated with pain and pleasure. Undoubtedly, the greatest part of human functions is performed on the pleasure level.

A crucial role in this issue must be assigned to the experiments in visceral conditioning (Bykov, 1957). These experimental studies have proved beyond doubt that the inner organs can respond with a pain–pleasure reaction. Apparently, pain and pleasure are not universal phenomena and probably start on a quite advanced level of biological evolution.

It seems, therefore, advisable to distinguish three evolutionary levels, namely the *prehedonic,* the *hedonic,* and the *posthedonic.* Evidently, conditioning processes can be conducted on any of the three levels, that is, the visceral prehedonic conditioning, the reward and punishment hedonic conditioning, and the posthedonic conditioning to be explained below. The prehedonic level corresponds to Ukhtomski's prepotence or shear-force conditioning (Razran, 1957).

Conditioning on the hedonic level is related to reward and punishment. I believe that there is also a third, post-hedonic level of conditioning. Certain functions of the human body are not accompanied by the feeling of pleasure as are other functions. For instance, the functions of division, growth, and decline of cells, the secretion of thyroxine, the growth of hair and nails, the growth of bones and muscles and of tumors in their initial stage are usually not accompanied by pleasure or pain. They are prehedonic. On the other hand, the secretion of semen, sucking, eating and drinking, rhythmical movements, overcoming obstacles, singing, and hugging and kissing are usually accompanied by pleasure. Deprivation of food is painful; deprivation of certain nutritional values may become ultimately dangerous for the organism, yet it is not painful, at least in its beginning. Thus pleasure applies to a certain part of human actions; some actions are guided by prepleasure or postpleasure factors that will be explained below.

There have been several instances when men acted in disregard of pain and pleasure. When a tired mother gets up in the middle of the night to take care of an infant, she certainly does not follow her wishes for comfort and pleasure. Restful sleep is definitely more enjoyable than sleepless nights spent at the crib of a sick child. When hungry parents give away the last piece of bread to their infants, they renounce pleasure and accept pangs of hunger willingly. Most parents will go into fire to save the lives of their children. Most people will do it for their friends; some will do it for strangers, for any human being in distress, as the history of the Danish resistance to the Nazis has proven.

History is full of examples of men and women who acted in an apparent renunciation of pleasure and disregard of pain. The early Christians did not seek escape from the Roman persecutions, and sang "Hallelujah" while being burned alive or thrown into cages of wild beasts. If avoidance of pain and pursuit of pleasure were the only motives of human actions, there would be no Christianity today, or Judaism either. In the wars of the little Judea against the Roman emperors, the Jewish people displayed utter disregard for pain and death.

In medieval and contemporary times, the Jewish people have been exposed to discrimination, hatred, and persecution. The persecutors, be it the Crusaders, the flagellants, the Christian kings, or the Holy Inquisition, gave the Jews the choice of either conversion to Christianity with all its privileges and joys or terrible persecution and torture for those Jews who remained faithful to the religion of their fathers. Some Jews could not reject pleasure and withstand pain. Most of them, however, made the choice and proudly refused to surrender. The heroic story of the Warsaw ghetto's fight in 1943 against the Nazis is symbolic of the history of mankind; the history of religious, national, and social movements knows many cases of self-sacrifice, courage, willing martyrdom, and heroism. Men and women have been willing to accept deprivation and pain, and refused to renounce or betray their friends, families, country, and ideals. An unconditional avoidance of pain and search for pleasure would render loyalty, honor, heroism, and ethics absolutely impossible.

Can pain be overcome?

> Pain may be decreased and even completely inhibited by psychological procedures, such as hypnosis, suggestion, and distraction. The most convincing cases are those in which major operations and obstetrical deliveries have been performed under hypnosis. Other patients have had amputations performed while praying to religious images and have said they felt no pain. Simple suggestion by the giving of placebos frequently reduces ordinary pain to a remarkable degree. Distraction by arousing

interest in things not connected with pain can be extraor-
dinarily effective. (Cobb, 1958, p. 288)

Cobb quotes Beecher's controlled experiments with graded
stimulation to nerve endings. Beecher and others concluded
that the extent of a wound bears only slight relationship to
the pain experienced. Cobb wrote, "A wound is not alone the
cause of pain; the significance of the wound may be the
paramount factor in determining the production of pain"
(1958, p. 288).

Bykov (1957, p. 339ff) reported a series of experiments
conducted by Pshonik. These experiments were devoted to
the study of the cortical dependence of pain reception and the
interconnection existing between the pain and heat reception.
Pain was caused by pricks of a needle and by the application
of heat (63 °C) to the skin. In preliminary experiments the
pain lasted for 10 seconds and resulted in vascular constriction
and, consequently, a fall of the plethysmogram. The plethysmogram has been used by research workers as an objective
measurement of pain.

Some experiments threw light on what Bykov named
"psychogenic pain." Pshonik applied 20 different combinations of bell and temperature below that of the pain stimulation and elicited in his subjects "the same vaso-constriction (a
fall of the plethysmogram) and the same subjective pain
sensations as the usual pain combinations of the bell and 63°"
(Bykov, 1957, p. 341). The conditioned stimulus, the bell, "trans-
forms a subdolorific stimulation into a pain stimulation."

In some experiments the unconditioned stimulus gave
zero on the plethysmogram, but the conditioned stimulus (a
combination of a tactile stimulus with the bell) changed the
effect of the unconditioned stimulus and evoked a constriction
of the vessels, and when applied with light evoked dilation.
Even words or speech signals of the second order evoked

more intense pain or pain inhibition reactions than unconditioned stimuli.

THE ANTIGONE PRINCIPLE

There are, apparently, human actions when the pain–pleasure consideration seems to disappear, or at least to become weaker. Bykov reported cases of wounded men who controlled their own pain. An analysis of vectorial attitudes shows that certain individuals are capable of suffering for the sake of others and sacrificing themselves to make others happy. The prototype of this attitude is parenthood or the willingness to give without taking.

Let us call this attitude the *Antigone principle,* after Antigone, the daughter of King Oedipus. When Oedipus left Thebes, his two sons started a fight and one was killed. The new king forbade the burial of the body of the fratricidal brother. In accordance with the Greek religion, the refusal to bury meant eternal suffering of the soul. Antigone decided to save her brother's soul and to bury him knowing very well that the king would impose capital punishment. This willingness to sacrifice one's own life for the beloved person or ideal is the Antigone principle (Wolman, 1965).

History is a huge and unsurpassed psychological laboratory. History bears witness not only to human actions guided by pleasure and pain, but it is full of actions of people who made history by their unrelentless pursuit of truth, such as Galileo, or social justice, such as Johann Huss. Thousands of fighters for freedom of conscience, whether persecuted by religious or secular authorities or tortured in dungeons or burned alive, defended their convictions with an utter disregard of pain and pleasure.

During the Israel War of Independence against the Arab invasion in 1948, I had the opportunity to interview several Israeli men and women who, exposed to grave dangers in isolated outposts and outnumbered by the invading hordes, were wounded in combat. Some of them performed acts of superb heroism. Even when hit by shells, badly bleeding, and severely injured, they protected their comrades, fighting despite pain and risking their own lives to save others. There was neither jubilance nor self-praise in their statements.

Most of them complained of inadequate supplies or poor equipment as well as the unfairness of a war of a few against so many. When asked about their wounds and sufferings, they said that they were fully aware of the wounds and did their best to stop the bleeding, but they had very little, if any, memory of pain, as if pain were suspended at the time of combat. Once they had returned from behind the front lines, they did moan with pain. When asked about their heroic deeds, they explained that what they had done was the only thing for them to do. How could they let their friends down? Or how could they let a precious piece of equipment fall into the enemy's hands? How could they run for life and let the enemies conquer the village to plunder, torture, murder, and mutilate its inhabitants?

Their stories had one common denominator: the feeling of duty and moral responsibility. It seemed that every single Israeli warrior carried the responsibility for the entire Israeli Army, the whole of Israel, and the entire past history of the Jewish people. The pain of one individual seemed to shrink or even disappear in face of the individual's commitment toward his or her group, faith, homeland, and moral convictions.

This vectorial commitment can be directed toward one's friends or children, one's country or religion, or one's moral and political convictions. It is the vectorial attitude, the attitude of unconditional giving without asking anything in return. Its prototype is parental love and devotion. A loving parent may not be aware of his or her own pain while he or she tries to alleviate that of the suffering child. A loving person willingly renounces his or her own pleasures when the happiness of the beloved is at stake.

The Antigone principle can be directed toward friends, lovers, or members of one's group; it can be objectified and directed toward religion, political philosophy, or science. Some people are capable of sacrificing themselves for their religious, political, or scientific beliefs and of renouncing pleasure and disregarding pain. They are able to function on a posthedonic level and their actions are guided by the Antigone principle.

The theory of interindividual cathexes offers a hypothetical explanation of the reduction of pain and pleasure. Giving is an expression of abundant object cathexis and, therefore, of a lowered self-cathexis. In schizophrenics little libido is cathected in their own organism and they tend not to be narcissistic; as a result, they are less sensitive to pain and pleasure (Cobb, 1958). Small wonder that narcissistic sociopaths who love no one except themselves are exceedingly sensitive to pain and tend to be hypochondriacs (Wolman, 1987).

LUST FOR LIFE: EROS AND ARES

To survive is the basic motive of all animal and human behavior, and the fight for survival dominates and precedes all other and any other animal and human actions. *Lust for Life* is the main driving force of all living organisms.

The process of life is a process of oxidation, digestion, incorporation, metabolism, and so on. The higher the species stands on the evolutionary ladder, the more complex its life processes are. Ultimately, the entire behavior of an organism is an aggressive–defensive process, for each organism either devours other organisms or protects itself by fight or flight against being devoured.

The basic, universal goal common to the entire animal world, including human beings, is *survival*. All actions of all living organisms are dominated by and directed toward this goal. Whatever they do, they do in order to stay alive. To eat and not to be eaten, this is the question. It is a question of life or death; life for the eater, death for the eaten up. Big fishes eat smaller fishes, and small fishes eat lesser fry.

Let us name this universal drive to stay alive lust for life. The lust for life is not the sole motive in animal and human behavior, but it certainly exercises final and irrevocable control over all other directions and aspects of behavior. Consider sex, curiosity, or play. A mortally wounded or starving organism has not the slightest inclination toward sexual behavior, nor would it engage in exploratory or playful activities.

Charles Darwin presented the issues of "good" and "bad" in a new light. All living creatures fight for survival. The concepts of good and evil are man-made value judgments; biology has no part in them. Survival of the fittest is the law of nature, and the natural state is neither Ovid's nor Jean Jacques Rousseau's "golden era" of peace and brotherhood, but rather Thomas Hobbes's *bellum omnium contra omnes* ("war of all against all"). Value judgments are a human prerogative; nature knows none of them.

It was under Darwin's influence that modern psychologists became interested in how organisms live and act and stay alive. MacDougall, Watson, Sechenov, and Pavlov were Darwin's disciples, as was Freud. Life and death became the subject matter of psychology. Psychologists gave up the discussion of how men were *supposed* to feel, think, and act, and began to study how men *do* feel, think, and act, and how they live and fight for survival.

The issues of life and death are inescapably connected with love and hate. There are obvious reasons for such a combination in human minds, for love means support of life and hatred leads to its destruction. God creates, Satan destroys. Those who love and create are called good; those who hate and destroy are called evil. Freud's theory of Eros and Thanatos closely corresponds to this antinomy of life and love versus death and hatred.

The difficulty with this otherwise plausible set of concepts lies in the lack of clarity regarding intraindividual and interindividual motives. Freud's death instinct is primarily suicidal in relation to the narcissistic direction of libido. Certainly, in phylo- and ontogenetic development libido is primarily narcissistic. Is destrudo also self-directed and thus a death-promoting energy?

Freud's own reasoning does not support the idea of this kind of death instinct. Reading Freud strengthens the belief that object-destrudo of the fight for survival is the sole source of hostility (Pribram and Gill, 1966).

> From the earliest times it was muscular strength which decided who owned things or whose will shall prevail. Muscular strength was soon supplemented by the use of tools; the winner was the one who had the better weapons or who used them the more skillfully. From the moment at which weapons were introduced, intellectual superiority already began to replace brute muscular strength but the final purpose of the fight remained the same. (Freud, 1933, pp. 274–275).

The killing of enemies has had two advantages: a dead enemy could not fight back and his ill fate deterred others.

An enemy's life could be spared whenever he could be forced into slave labor or when his broken might represented no threat to the victor. In times when physical forces counted most, men were killed, but women and children were included in the spoil.

The following hypothetical system is introduced: Every living organism carries a certain amount of energy. This energy is activated by threats to one's life. The built-in release apparatus, the force that opens the valves of the hydraulic model, is called instinctual drive.

This force activates energies in the direction of survival. Thus it should be named "lust for life." At a certain evolutionary level part of this energy became invested in procreation or the preservation of the life of the species as if the life of one individual continued through his offspring.

Life and death of a single organism are terms that indicate the viability of the organism. There are degrees of viability. An organism can be forceful, full of energy, most capable of providing food for itself, and well prepared for self-defense. Or it may be sick, declining, and dwindling to nothing. When the vital energies become exhausted and vitality reaches the zero point, the organism dies. Lack of lust for life does not point to self-destructive tendencies; it is precisely what it is, namely, a decline in the zest for life. An organism that has lost its urge to live may give up the fight for survival and die.

As long as an organism is alive, its energies can be used in two directions, either toward the promotion of life or toward its destruction. The instinctual force, lust for life, divides into two arms, the one that serves promotion of life is Eros or love. Love can be directed toward oneself or toward others. The other arm serves destruction and may be called Ares. Ares, too, can be directed toward oneself or toward others. Life and death deal with *quantities* of energy; the terms "love" and "hostility" indicate the *direction* in which mental energy is used by Eros and Ares.

There is but one general universal drive, the lust for life. There is, for organisms, only one general biochemical energy. But the energy can be transformed into mental energy in a transitionistic fashion and the discharge of energy can go in either direction. It is Eros and libido whenever it supports life; libido can be invested in oneself or in others, in a sexual or a desexualized way. Whenever there is a threat to life, the self-directed Eros is accompanied by the object-directed Ares.

Ares is the name for the destructive arm of the universal lust for life drive and serves the same purpose of survival as Eros does. Should an immortal and omnipotent creature exist whose life could never have been threatened, however, such a creature would be pure Eros; such a creature would have had no use for Ares.

But all living organisms, including human beings, live under the threat of inanimate and animate nature. To fact this threat, lust for life turns not into Eros, but into Ares. Eros and Ares are two channels of the same drive of lust for life; activated in two different types of situations, they serve basically the same goal, the survival of the individual, and, in some situations, survival of the species.

It seems that Ares is not only a more primitive and phylogenetically earlier drive than Eros, but as a rule it is more powerful than Eros. Pavlov's dogs did not copulate when their skin was burned, but the salivated even when he burnt their skin (Pavlov, 1928, p. 228). The cortical food center is stronger than the skin center and the sex center is weaker than the skin center. When Pavlov tried to crush the dog's bones, even salivation stopped. Hungry dogs can bear minor wounds, but bone breaking means death, and in face of death all energy is mobilized for self-defense.

Hungry, thirsty, sick, and wounded organisms act in an aggressive and destructive manner (Hamburg and Trudeau, 1981). It seems that whenever the supply of libido is used up, the organism works on destrudo. Libido seems to be a "higher" fuel, destrudo a "lower" one; when there is no immediate threat to life, a balanced love for oneself and for others may suffice for survival. In emergencies the destrudo takes over, and in danger and anger people act with what seems to be added energy, the latent energy of destrudo.

Eros and Ares are the two basic releasers of mental energy. Ares, like Eros, has an impetus, source, object, and aim. The impetus is the amount of destructive energy (destrudo) that is discharged. Its source is a threat to one's own life. The aim of Ares is the complete or partial destruction of enemies. The object can be oneself or another organism.

The somatic changes in Ares are accelerated heart beat, perspiration, trembling, contraction of muscles, baring of teeth, growling, and so on. The threat of annihilation is the main cause of the somatic changes. The hostile action, which is a discharge of destrudo aiming at the destruction of the threatening object, restores the inner balance (analogous with the actions of Eros). The threat may be related to an inner stimulus of hunger or an outer stimulus that jeopardizes one's life, prevents satisfaction of hunger, prevents escape, or any other combination of hostile stimuli.

Pavlov (1928, p. 255ff) believed that hostile behavior is a guarding reaction against real or threatened injury. Experimental studies on frustration stressed the fact that frustrated individuals tend to become hostile. It seems, however, that any adverse life condition and any threat may act as a releaser of hostile behavior. Antisocial actions are multiple and diversified, including persecution of minorities or any other type of violence (Hamburg and Trudeau, 1981; Keith, 1984).

Most often aggressive behavior originates in the fear that one's life is threatened. Usually people do not hate unless they fear. Immortals do not have to fight for survival; an omniscient and omnipotent being does not hate. Buddha did not hate. Nor did Jesus. Only the perfect and immortal being can forgive all his enemies because he does not fear them.

But animals and human beings fear death and hate their enemies because enemies inflict injury that may kill them. The strongest fear is the mortal fear, the fear of perishing, the fear of losing what all people have: life.

DESTRUDO

Nothing could be farther from truth than the belief that humans are basically kind and loving beings. Even a cursory perusal of history adduces convincing evidence of human belligerence. All human societies, starting with the cavemen through the generations of warriors, conquerors, tyrants, and henchmen have displayed a never-ending series of offensive and defensive, holy and unholy wars. All human beings are motivated by the fundamental urge to stay alive, the lust for life. "To eat and not to be eaten" is the guiding principle of human behavior, and the fight for survival is the main concern of *all* human beings.

I have introduced the name of the Greek god of war Ares as a symbol of readiness to fight for survival. The Aretic, that is, the belligerent offensive–defensive actions dominate human behavior. These actions activate the major part of human energies, and Aretic motivation is the chief releaser of energy. Threats to one's life make one more energetic than ever, and dangerous situations activate hitherto unused resources.

Destrudo will be therefore the appropriate name for the mental energies used to destroy whatever we need for food and those who want to use us for their food. It seems methodologically advisable to hypothesize that a threat to life is most likely to activate the maximum of energy stored in an organism. Ferocious beasts use very little energy unless they are hungry and attack the prey, or when they are attacked and may fall prey.

Something similar happens to human beings. The presumably kind, friendly, God-loving, mild-mannered person who hardly does anything at all can easily become vociferous and bursting with energy whenever faced with a real or imaginary threat to his or her life or self-esteem. Just try to attack him, contradict him, or make a disparaging remark about him or his God and the loving, good man or woman will turn into a vicious predator.

All living organisms practice defensive–offensive behavior. They defend themselves against those who want to eat them and attack those they want to eat. Aggressive, destructive, belligerent, violent behavior directed toward those who want to destroy you or those you want to destroy is the motive of all behavior common to all living organisms. All living organisms are belligerent. All kill to eat, and all kill in order not to be devoured. (Hamburg and Trudeau, 1981; Bandura, 1973).

FOUR TYPES OF HOSTILE BEHAVIOR

The first type of hostile behavior is aggressive and the second defensive; both are directly related to self-protection. In the *aggressive* type the wolf acts in a hostile manner toward the sheep by virtue of its intention to eat it. No feeling of hate is involved in eating unless the sheep resists. Men who eat chicken do not hate chickens but nonetheless destroy them. The instinctual source of aggressive hostility is the threat of starvation. Hungry beasts attack.

The second type of hostility is *defensive;* it is usually combined with hate. Defensive hostility is aimed at the destruction of a deadly menace. It leads sheep to fight against wolves and man to fight against enemies and predatory animals. It is reflected in a child's fight against another child who hits him or takes away his toy. Defensive hostility aims at the destruction of the forces that jeopardize survival. One may defend himself by fight or flight, but he hates in either case.

Other types of hostility serve survival in a less efficient manner. The third type, *panic,* implies an impulsive, unplanned, often useless effort to escape danger. People caught in fire may push one another against locked doors instead of rationally seeking exit. There is neither consideration nor mutual help in panic; goats chased by wolves fight one another, overcrowding and blocking the narrow escape passages.

The fourth type of hostility, *terror,* can be seen in mortally wounded animals who attack indiscriminately. Because no gain can be expected from turning blindly against everything, terror must be considered as pure Ares gone wild in the face of a lethal danger.

Hostile actions can be repressed or displaced, just as libidinal actions are. Hate can be displaced from the menacing object to some other object and turned into scapegoatism. Destrudo may turn not against the real cause of damage but against one's own ego in a self-defeating or self-destructive manner. Destrudo can be combined with libido and turned into sadism. When rationalized, it assumes the proportions of fanaticism and chauvinism; when sufficiently kindled they result in wars.

Ares, like Eros, can undergo innumerable changes. It starts as a defense against dangers combined with self-directed Eros. But it may become hate without danger, cruelty without gain, cruelty combined with sexual pleasure, or hate for oneself. As mentioned earlier, discharge of the aggressive energy (destrudo) is as pleasurable as any other discharge of instinctual energy.

Consider the story of the Vandals. After looting the treasures of Rome, they demolished whatever they could not carry away with them. During World War I, the Germans plundered, tortured, and murdered the Belgians without apparent reason. Destrudo can be acted out for the sheer pleasure of vandalism.

Lorenz (1966) once said that "the presence of an outlet for an external aggression is necessary to prevent intramarital fighting" (p. 73). The history of persecutions and wars, especially the history of Nazi Germany, bear unmistakable witness to the brutal force of Ares. Although Ares starts as a self-defensive device, it may become a goal in itself. Men may derive great satisfaction from a display of violent force. The discharge of destructive energy create a feeling of power, thus magnifying one's self-confidence. Screaming at and hitting someone makes one feel strong and thus enhances one's estimate of one's own vitality.

Depression and elation are emotional corollaries of perceiving oneself as weak or strong, respectively. Depression is the feeling of helpless anger directed against oneself and others. Elation is an expression of an abundant feeling of power. Manic-depressive patients in a manic phase are full of love for themselves and others, in depression they hate everybody including themselves (Wolman and Stricker, 1990).

POWER

Every human being has some amount of power, whether it is physical, mental, political, financial, or any other. Power is the ability to satisfy needs, and survival is the common name of all needs. In order to survive, people need oxygen, water, food, shelter, protection against enemies, and so on. The more power people have, the better are their chances for survival. Some people use power beyond the fundamental biological needs, and they follow their personal ambitions, desires, and whims.

The more one is aware of the extent and limitation of his power, the better use he can make of his resources. People who overestimate their own power take unnecessary and costly risks; those who underestimate do not try to do what they could safely do.

One can increase his power either by himself or with outside help. The simplest way is to improve one's physical fitness, muscular strength, and agility. Power has always attracted people, and all children and adults are fascinated by the stories of Samson and Hercules, Mighty Mouse and Superman.

As humanity has grown older, cunning and weaponry have become the main source of power and feeling of security. Weapons are expensive, and in contemporary society power is most often related to economic resources. Many people strive to political power, leadership, and control of others, and history is full of men (and women) who strove to accumulate political power, possessions, and glory.

Apparently, the desire to be strong is universal, and people derive a great deal of the feeling of security that is synonymous with the feeling of power. However, no human being is so powerful as to be able to overcome all threats, and no one, except maniacs, drunkards, and drug addicts, believes in his own omnipotence. The painful feeling of weakness leads some people to seek the morbid and harmful escape of alcohol and drugs. Well-adjusted individuals put all their efforts to increase their real power and security, which is awareness of their power.

There are two rational methods of increasing one's power. One is by the growth of one's own power, the other by forming alliances. Both methods increase one's chances for survival. The first method implies depending on one's own resources, and the second, depending on others. One's power and feeling of security can be substantially increased through interaction with other people.

Interaction with other people, however, is not always conducive to security. People react to situations in accordance with their own perception, that is, not the way things are but the way they see things. One seeks help from a dentist whom he perceives as strong, that is, competent and capable of taking care of the teeth, and friendly, that is, willing to do it, honest, and caring. One would not go to a dentist perceived as a weak, that is, incompetent, nor to one perceived as being hostile, that is, deceitful.

Human relations are determined by power (the ability to satisfy needs) and acceptance (willingness to do so or to prevent it), as perceived. There are four determinants of human relations, two related to power, namely, strong or weak, and two related to acceptance, namely, friendly or hostile.

There are four possible combinations of perceiving people as strong, weak, friendly, or hostile, as follows: (1) strong and friendly, (2) strong and hostile, (3) weak and friendly, or (4) weak and hostile.

People perceived as being strong and friendly elicit the desire to be associated with them. People choose them and follow them for they are trusted (acceptance) and depended on (power). People tend to cooperate with them and do not wish to lose their valuable friendship.

People perceived as being strong but hostile evoke fear and hatred. One avoids them and waits for the opportunity to hurt them.

Friendly but weak people elicit pity. No one respects them nor does one car for their friendship and approval. One may feel sorry for them and tend to help them, but one has no respect for them nor does one seek to be associated with them.

Weak and hostile people evoke disgust and hatred.

In summary, there are two main sources of security: (1) one's own power, and (2) the power of dependable allies (acceptance).

The awareness of one's power is *self-confidence* and *self-reliance*. The awareness of having strong and friendly allies is trust. Self-confidence and trust are the two main ingredients in the feeling of security.

Social Relations as a Function of Power and Acceptance

Eros and Ares are theoretical constructs introduced in an isomorphic manner to the observable positive and negative uses of power. These theoretical constructs may serve as a useful link between Freud's depth psychology and observational and experimental data.

People tend to view themselves and others in the dimensions of power and acceptance. The amount of power (what one can do) depends on one's ability to satisfy his own needs and the needs of others. Acceptance (what one is willing to do for someone) indicates the direction in which power is used, either for the satisfaction of needs and protection of life (Eros) or for the prevention of need satisfaction and destruction of life (Ares), either of oneself (self-directed) or others (object-directed).

Assuming that survival is the main motive of human behavior, its chief corollary is the drive for power. Being mortal and vulnerable, people tend to increase their own power (that is, their chances for survival) through association with other people. Naturally, one seeks to associate with friendly people, that is, those who use their power in the defense of his life, and, obviously, one wishes his friends to be strong. In other words, people prefer to associate with those who are strong and friendly.

Fromm (1941, p. 24) maintained that the Middle Ages were an era of security based on strong intragroup ties and solidarity. Within the framework of the feudal system each social class offered a powerful support and gave its members the feeling of power derived from group solidarity. The power of any given individual was enhanced by his class belonging.

Belonging to a group, however, does not necessarily guarantee friendly relations among the members of a group. People form groups for a variety of reasons, and they may relate to the other members in more than one way.

Some people join a group in order to have their own needs satisfied; they have in mind taking and not giving. They join a group only for their own benefit and pursue their own objectives; they belong to a group because without the group they could not satisfy their needs or they would have encountered considerable difficulties. Whenever the particular relationship or the particular group ceases to satisfy their needs, they will leave it.

This kind of a group, called instrumental, represents the usual business relationship. When a man looks for a job or starts a business, he enters an instrumental social relationship and his objective is to receive remuneration or profit. The employer's attitude is instrumental also, for the only thing he wants is to find a man to help him in his trade. A shopkeeper wants to sell his goods to a customer not because he wants to supply the customer, but for a profit; it is an instrumental relationship—the shopkeeper wants to satisfy his own needs.

Apparently people form instrumental groups because otherwise their needs could not be satisfied. Sociability in human beings starts out of weakness and the instrumental attitude bears witness to that. A new organism starts life dependent on the organism that gave life; the intrauterine life is a parasitic process of taking without giving anything in return. This parasitic, taking attitude continues in infancy: the infant is a taker and the parents or parental substitutes are the givers. The infant is too weak to give; he must receive all the necessary supplies or he will not survive. Also, a drowning man who calls for help is instrumental.

During the first two years, the child learns to love others. According to Montagu (1962), some people become symbols of satisfaction because they provide the child with the means of satisfaction.

Maturation and learning processes are well illustrated by the growth of the infant's power, that is, the ability to satisfy his or her own needs. The infant becomes capable of such things as maintaining balance, walking, grasping, and holding things.

The first social contacts of the infant are the supporting and protecting adults. As soon as the infant meets other children, the situation changes. Adults were the givers, he was the taker, but peers are takers just as he is. To become a giver, one has to be assured about his possessions. The child must feel quite self-confident to be ready to face other children.

The more help, the more love and affection the child has received, the more he is sure of forthcoming help. The more he feels secure and protected, the sooner he will develop the feeling of self-confidence. In terms of the power and acceptance theory, the friendly and supportive attitude of parents gives the child an increasing feeling of his own power and enables him to enter the higher developmental stage of give-and-take mutual relationships. An anxious, insecure child may be afraid of other children and have difficulties in relating to them on a give-and-take basis.

Several factors help the child arrive at the mutual level of a voluntary give-and-take relationship. The first factor is the child's own growth and learning that lead toward an increasing mastery of his own body and acquisition of skills. Success is a good therapist; it helps to build one's self-confidence.

The second factor is his undisturbed instrumental relationship with parental figures and other relevant adults. Several workers have observed the importance of parental approval for the development of the child's self-confidence (e.g., Adler, Horney, Sullivan). Parental acceptance and approval is the very foundation for the child's feeling of security, and the more the child is sure of continuous parental support, the more courage he will have in forming social relations with peers on a give-and-take basis.

The third factor is the interaction with peers, the rewarding experience of sharing, trading, taking turns, and helping each other. Children who are rejected by their peers and assaulted or ridiculed may regress into a defensive guarding attitude of withdrawal and hostility. The simple fact of being among children does not necessarily encourage social development. Children may reject, hurt, and humiliate a shy and withdrawn child. The misfortunes in group living may set development back and force more withdrawal and more world-destructive, revengeful fantasies.

In mutual relations the desire to give, to be friendly, and to accept the other person comes to the fore. This relationship is based on the fact that both parties have the same desire to give. The instrumental relationship may entail some giving also; the employee who looks for a job to earn his living *must* give his work. But this is not his objective, and my division of social relations is based on the objectives of the participants.

In a mutual relationship, the aim is to give and to receive. Hence there is love in them, love being defined as willingness to be of help. In instrumental relationships there is the desire to receive love but not to give it. In mutual relations there is the desire to give and to receive.

When one feels weak, he is inclined to seek help; he wants to get support to make himself stronger and to increase his chances for survival. Poor men beg, hungry wolves attack. Children born during economic depressions, who are brought up in deprivation, tend to be acquisitive and greedy. These types of behavior can be hostile or not, but all of them are acquisitive.

Obviously, it takes both development and learning to become capable of self-sacrifice and of giving without asking anything in return. A little child is selfish, instrumental, willing to take, because the child is weak and needs support. As he grows and becomes stronger, he becomes more and more capable of sharing and of mutual relations.

Parenthood is the prototype of vectorialism. Parents create life, protect it, and care for it irrespective of their child's looks, health, IQ, disposition, and success. The weaker the child, the more they must protect it. The more the infant needs their help, the more sympathy he should elicit in them.

No human being can be vectorial all the time. Some human beings may never develop a vectorial attitude, while some others develop it frequently and to a great extent. And yet the most fatherly or motherly or self-sacrificing and saintly individuals, when exposed to a lethal danger, may slide down to instrumentalism and call desperately for help. Or, in black despair, they may sink below instrumentalism into the hateful rage of a wounded animal.

Normal human beings are capable of functioning adequately in all three types of social relations, and can be instrumental in business, mutual in marriage, and vectorial in parenthood. One may also combine some of these attitudes in a rational manner, and in certain situations reach the Antigone level, which is the peak of vectorialism (Wolman, 1982).

FEAR AND ANGER

Threats to one's life or to one's security incite one to fight or flight. In most mammals a threat provokes an attack on the source of threat. Hunger, no escape routes, and familiarity with the territory encourage defensive aggression. Very young, very old, and sick animals tend to escape.

A threat to human beings evokes fear or anger or both, depending on how one perceives the source of threat. Strong and hostile enemies elicit more fear, weak and hostile ones more anger. Fear and anger are two sides of the same coin of self-preservation. One reacts more with fear when one believes that the threatening forces are overwhelming. One reacts more in anger when one feels he could defeat the hostile forces. Usually people react with both fear and anger, but are rarely angry at those they do not fear at all.

Both fear and anger are hostile stimuli. The weaker one is, the more reasons for fear and anger. A self-assured mother does not fear or get angry at a cranky and difficult child because he does not represent a threat to her. She calms him down by her self-assured and friendly attitude, for the stronger she is, the less she fears and the less angry she is.

FEAR AND PERCEPTION

As mentioned previously, human behavior is guided not by things as they are but as they are seen. People may possess a great deal of power and have many powerful friends and be unaware of all that. Power and acceptance as perceived by the individual are the main determinants of behavior. An individual who is aware of his own power and of his allies is reasonably well prepared to cope with dangers.

An overestimation of one's own resources combined with underestimation of the potential threat may lead to a maladjustive lack of fear, and hyperoptimistic and overconfident attitude may bring self-defeat.

Fear is a normal reaction that helps survival provided it is *realistic* and based on a correct estimate of the potential threat and the power one possesses himself and the dependability of one's allies. Fear is adjustive if it corresponds to the real situation.

Fear is rational when it is based on the awareness of overwhelming threats; it is irrational when one overestimates the power of the threatening forces and/or underestimates his own powers. Overestimation of one's own powers makes one vulnerable, but underestimation of one's power makes one fear nonexisting dangers.

Acute states of fear create morbid physiological reactions such as trembling, profuse perspiration, faint feelings, weakness in joints and muscles, nausea, diarrhea, and disturbances in motor coordination. A frightened individual may seek escape when none is needed.

Unrealistic, irrational fears can have a crippling effect on human behavior. People obsessed by irrational fears are unable to use their resources and defend themselves even against enemies.

Severe states of fear often cause regressive phenomena in adults as well as in children. During World War II, I had the opportunity to see panic-driven adults who temporarily lost control of bowel and bladder and regressed to baby talk. Severe fears adversely affected their insight and foresight and impaired judgment and self-control.

The regressive phenomena are even more dangerous in children who have not had the chance to develop a mature personality structure as described in the book *Children without Childhood* (Wolman, 1970). The younger the child, the more damage can be caused to his or her personality.

ANXIETY

The terms "fear" and "anxiety" are often used interchangeably. It might, however, be useful to introduce a clear distinction between these terms. The physiological reactions of fear and anxiety are quite similar and involve the reaction of the sympathetic part of the autonomic nervous system. They adversely affect the gastrointestinal system, increase the secretion of adrenaline, speed up the heart rate, and so on. However, fear is a reaction to a specific real or unreal danger, such as fear of vicious dogs, burglars, and kidnappers. The term *anxiety* denotes a widespread gloomy feeling of impending doom.

Fear is a momentary reaction to danger. It is based on a low estimate of one's own power compared with the power of the threatening factors. A fear disappears with the change of balance of power. The disappearance of the threatening person, animal, or object puts an end to the fear. Also, a change in one's estimate of his own power in comparison to the danger removes fear.

Anxiety is a feeling of one's overall weakness, ineptness, and helplessness. Anxiety is tantamount to the loss of self-esteem. Expecting impending doom, an anxious individual may withdraw from usual activities and become irritable and unproductive. Anxiety may also, albeit temporarily, affect one's intellectual function. Anxiety may make one momentarily forget things he knows, stutter or stammer, and be unable to communicate his thoughts.

Anxiety implies an overall feeling of one's own weakness and one's inability to cope with dangers. An anxious individual underestimates his ability to cope with life in general. The presence of dependable allies and the familiarity with a threatening situation do not allay one's anxiety. Anxiety does not come from without; it comes from the unconscious, from within.

COURAGE

Courage implies faith in one's self and self-reliance and self-confidence. Courage is the feeling that one has enough *power* to stand up and be counted.

Genuine courage is realistic. It is closely related to a correct estimate of one's own power and the power of the threatening enemies. Courageous men and women take all the necessary precautions and use all their resources in order to win. Self-defeating individuals who overlook unsurmountable odds and throw themselves into dangerous situations are desperados. They do not display courage but self-destructive behavior.

The degree of courage depends on a variety of factors, and the same individual may act differently in different situations. Poor physical health makes one feel weak, and in many but not all cases it adversely affects one's courage. Group involvement and the sense of commitment to people or to an idea, self-respect, and feeling of responsibility are highly relevant ingredients of courage.

Loneliness usually reduces one's courage. The presence of people perceived as strong and friendly, that is, having power and willing to help, greatly enhances one's courage. Most people display much more courage when they take part in a group action. Large numbers of people can dull one's sense of reality and awareness of dangers, however, and mob behavior may be more brazen than courageous.

SECURITY

As previously stated, the basic need of all human beings is to stay alive. The feeling of one's own strength is the emotional corollary of this need. This feeling can be derived from one's own ability to provide food, water, shelter, and protection against hostile forces (power) and/or of dependence on one's strong and friendly allies (acceptance). The awareness of one's own resources creates the feeling of self-reliance; the awareness of dependable allies gives rise to the feeling of trust.

Horney, Sullivan, Fromm, and other sociologically oriented neoanalysts have stressed the feeling of security derived from childhood experience. In most cases the feeling of security originates in support that comes from without, and it is a continuous lifelong process of ups and downs, depending on interindividual balance of power and the individual's perception of this balance.

The feeling of security can be described as follows: The individual is convinced that he is able to provide the food, water, and shelter he needs as well as stand up to hostile men, animals, and forces of nature. He also believes that in danger he can count on help from without. In childhood the dependence on others is the main factor in security. In adulthood self-reliance plays the major role. At all times the feeling of security is a combination of both, except in pathological cases of depressive and manic moods to be described later on.

The feeling of power derived from within (self-reliance) and without (trust) branches off into several avenues. The need to feel strong serves as a basic ingredient in several aspects of human nature, but it would be an oversimplification to reduce the entire human motivation to a single need.

INTERINDIVIDUAL DIFFERENCES

There are several motivational factors somewhat related to power and acceptance (Krauss and Krauss, 1977). Although each motive can be described as an independent factor, all motives are often mutually interrelated and, as a rule, intertwined with the main motives of survival and security.

Maslow (1968) suggested the following hierarchy of needs or drives in order of declining universality. Physiological needs are universal, common to all human beings. Next come safety needs, then belongingness and love, then esteem, and finally, the least common need is the need for self-actualization.

My contention is that these needs are universal and they are present in every human being to a certain degree. The intraindividual balance of drives and needs is typical for every individual, and the difference in intensity and hierarchy of needs within every personality accounts for interindividual differences. To use a figurative presentation, every personality is comprised of the same elements, but there are substantial differences in quantity and organization of these elements. Some individuals have more of one element and less of

another, and there are significant interindividual differences
concerning the relative role a particular element plays in
behavior. For instance, just the degree of involvement with
other people, that is, the amount of interindividual cathexes
of libido and destrudo, is responsible for highly different
personality types and behavioral patterns. Innate abilities, life
experiences, and present environmental factors make every
individual different from anyone else despite the fact that all
human beings are basically cast in the same elements.

THE NEED TO BE ACCEPTED

It was mentioned above that despite diversity of motivational factors, the need to survive and its corollaries are the
common roots and highly significant ingredients of human
behavior. Let us follow Maslow's list. Physiological needs,
except for sex (to be discussed in the following chapter) are
clearly related to survival. The need for oxygen, food, water,
sleep, and so on are fundamental survival needs.

The need for security is clearly related to survival. There
are two basic reactions to a threat, namely fear and anger or
a combination of the two. Fear is a reaction based on a low
estimate of one's own strength and a high estimate of strength
of the threatening people, animals, or situation (Erikson, 1963;
Horney, 1939). Whenever fear is based on a correct evaluation
of one's own resources in comparison to the threats, the fear
has survival value and it is, therefore, an adjustive reaction.
When one overestimates the power of the threatening people,
animals, or situations and/or underestimates his own powers,
his fear is irrational and maladjustive. Anxiety was previously
defined as a general feeling of one's own weakness. A grave
underestimation of one's resources leads to depression and an
overestimation, that is, a highly exaggerated opinion of one's

powers combined with totally unrealistic underestimation of potential threats, leads to elation. As will be explained later, the entire gamut of mental or behavioral disorders (I am using the two terms interchangeably) is related to survival and its corollaries of power and acceptance.

Maslow's concept of love and belonging echoes Horney's and Sullivan's emphasis on the child's need to feel loved and accepted. According to Horney the need to feel loved and accepted and protected is the basic need in human life. A child who does not feel accepted by his parents develops what Horney called "basic anxiety." The unwanted, unloved, rejected child may feel "isolated and helpless in a potentially hostile world" (Horney, 1939).

Sullivan (1953) maintained that the child somehow dimly perceives or empathizes parental attitudes. As long as the child feels that he is accepted and loved, he develops the feeling of well-being and happiness, called *euphoria.* This euphoria disappears when the child who receives food feels rejected. Rejection produces feelings of insecurity, that is, anxiety.

There has been ample evidence that children desperately need to feel accepted and protected. The physical expressions of affection, such as cuddling, kissing, hugging, and pleasant words, enhance the child's feeling of security and promote his mental health.

A newborn child is helpless. He may not survive unless he receives adequate protection. His physical survival depends on meeting his basic needs, but his mental health greatly depends on his *trust* that his needs are willingly met and also will be met in the future.

As mentioned before, the child's growth and development gradually reduces his dependence on others. The role of trust in others (acceptance) is gradually reduced and the reliance on his own strength (power) increases. Adult men and women cannot be omnipotent, but the more they rely on themselves, the less they depend on outside support. Overdependence in adulthood is a sign of immaturity.

SELF-ESTEEM AND SELF-ACTUALIZATION

The need for esteem and self-actualization develop gradually, but they are always related to the fundamental lust for life drive.

The child's self-esteem originates in parental approval. Infants have no criteria for self-evaluation; they take parental communication seriously and uncritically accept parental pronounciations. I had in treatment young and attractive girls who believed themselves to be "ugly ducklings" because their parents said so. Many male patients of mine were anxiety-ridden underachievers because they were victimized by parental harsh criticism.

Self-esteem originates in esteem given by others. A child's self-esteem thrives on parental verbal and nonverbal signs of acceptance. A self-assured child tends to win peer approval and is less sensitive to potential setbacks and rejections by peers. Gradually his or her own achievements play an increasing role in self-esteem, and the solid self-confidence given by the parents prepares the child for taking in stride the inevitable failures and frustrations. Insecure people tend to become conformists and act, as the joke tells, by "buying things they don't need, for money they don't have, to please people they don't know." Self-esteem in mature adults does not depend on outside approval but on inner harmony between what one feels one is supposed to do (superego's demands) and what one could possibly have done

(ego's realistic appraisal). Approval by others is always wel-
come, but in mature adults it is relegated to a secondary place,
sort of a "fringe benefit."

What one is supposed to do and what realistically one
can do is perhaps the essence of satisfactory adjustment to
life. Life as a biological phenomenon has no intrinsic goal.
It is a process of birth, growth, decay, and death. The
only purpose, if any, of a living organism is to stay alive
and to protect oneself against illness, injury, and death. Ultimately, all this is futile, for all organisms face the same
inescapable end.

While the end of the journey is always the same, however, some people travel in broken cars on bumpy roads while
others have a magnificent journey. Human beings have no
choice concerning the beginning and the end of life, but it is
up to them to decide how to live, how to cope with hardships,
and how to make life meaningful to them.

People set goals for themselves and struggle to attain them. Achieving contributes to a feeling of self-
confidence and pride, which are corollaries to the feeling of
one's own power.

The choice of targets can be whimsical, irrational, imposed from without, and/or futile. People may aspire to
things that have no real value to them or are totally out
of reach.

A rational choice of goals is based on a correct estimate
of one's resources, which include innate abilities, acquired
skills, and so on. Human actions are not performed in a
vacuum, and a rational choice of targets must consider environmental factors and opportunities.

The term *self-actualization* implies an adequate use
of one's resources toward the attainment of realistic goals.
Realization of one's potentialities in whatever direction

they lead, be it economic success, science, art politics, and so on, gives the individual the feeling of fulfillment and self-esteem. One can enjoy many things, such as sex and food, good company and good music, but one feels happy when one's dreams come true. Victory, triumph, overcoming hardship, and attainment of one's goals are the true sources of happiness, which is, ultimately, the wonderful feeling of power (Adler, 1929; Horney, 1939; Maslow, 1968; Murphy, 1947; Rychlak, 1984).

4

Love, Sex, and Violence

BIOLOGICAL FACTORS

There is no doubt that the sexual urge in its intensity is second only to the lust for life. The basic needs, such as hunger and thirst, serve survival. Sex does not. The lack of food causes death, the lack of sex does not. The function of primary drives is survival; the functions of sex do not protect the individual but propagate the species.

The sexual drive is innate, common to all higher biological species that reproduce by copulation. In most biological species, however, sexual intercourse is not related to any feelings whatsoever. One can hardly ascribe emotions to sex in insects.

There is a clear-cut biological distinction in sex roles. One male is able to fertilize several females and pregnant females are the sole carriers of offspring.

Biological differences between the sexes are an undeniable fact. Reproductive organs, sexual desires, menstruation, pregnancy, childbirth, breast feeding, and menopause are not cultural artifacts; they are biological differences. However, there is no evidence that girls are born to be kind, considerate,

85

and caring and that boys are born competitive and belligerent. In human beings, the prenatal gonadal hormones do not determine future behavioral differences between boys and girls (Wolman and Money, 1980). Psychological and sociological gender identity is usually imprinted on boys and girls in their second and third year of life, and considerable patterns of gender-related behavior are acquired in childhood. However, no male can learn the biological rhythms and functions of female organisms.

The idea of male supremacy is far from being a proven fact. Since the inception of written history, this assumption had found many backers. One of the most quoted sources is the Bible, for the Lord Himself is believed to have said to Eve, "He shalt rule over thee."

PSYCHOLOGY OF WOMEN

One can hardly find significant scientific literature describing male psychology, while numerous volumes have been written about the psychology of women. Men seem to differ from one another, and their common gender cannot obliterate the differences in intelligence, emotionality, special talents, social attitudes, and so on. No psychologist or psychiatrist believes that all men share common psychological traits and act in a similar manner just because of their gender communality. Obviously, the same must apply to women. The gentle and brilliant Madame Marie Curie and the Auschwitz monster, Else Koch, were females. The Russian Empress Katherine the Second had more in common with the Czar Ivan the Terrible than with Mrs. Franklin Delano Roosevelt.

Helene Deutsch (1945) ascribed to women narcissistic features, passivity, and masochistic tendencies. However, there is no reason at all to assume that all or most women are narcissistic. Narcissistic personality traits are the outstanding feature of the antisocial sociopaths (I called them hyper-instrumental narcissistic types), men and women alike (Wolman, 1987).

> Sociopaths tend to believe that they are poor, innocent, hungry, lonely and mistreated creatures. They fear confrontations with equals but do not hesitate to attack those who appear defenseless. Male and female sociopaths are criminals at heart who will or will not commit a crime depending on the weakness of the victim and the danger involved in attack. Most sociopaths avoid antisocial acts for which they may be punished and when they are caught, they regret not the crime but the punishment.

The term passivity is rather ambiguous and thus open to a host of interpretations. Deutsch assumed that women wait for things to happen instead of forging ahead. Expecting instead of inviting, accepting instead of giving, are allegedly universal feminine traits. It seems, however, that these personality traits are typical for mentally retarded, senile cases, paralytics, and terminal tuberculotics of either gender. Average men and women are never totally passive, except when they are physically and/or mentally exhausted. The vast majority of human beings are actively pursuing the processes of life, seeking food and shelter, and so on. They may, in depression and despair, passively surrender to adverse conditions, but states of anxiety and depression are not limited to one sex only.

The thesis of feminine masochism does not hold much water either. Sexual and nonsexual masochistic behavior is indicative of definite pathology, and is not at all a typical behavioral pattern of women. Enjoying good food, pretty dresses, and nice apartments, looking for a successful marriage combined with emotional and financial security are certainly more common than a gloomy, masochistic search for suffering. Most hysterics and manic-depressives are psychological masochists, but this applies to both sexes.

For centuries, women were programmed to stay home and to take care of children, but child care is by no means a female monopoly. Among subhuman species, male hamadryas display a protective attitude toward their female partners and their offspring.

Williams (1977, p. 149) reported a study of nurturant behavior, as follows:

> Fathers and mothers of newborns were observed in the hospital. When the baby was brought in, the nurturant behavior, looking, holding, smiling, rocking, of each parent was observed. Except for smiling, fathers exhibited more such behavior than mothers did. When the parents were observed separately with the baby, fathers were at least as nurturant in their behavior as mothers were.

The Arapesh males and females in New Guinea have been described by Margaret Mead (1950) as friendly, cooperative, and considerate. Male and female children were brought up the same way, and adult men and women shared child care and household responsibilities.

Mead did not find significant behavioral differences between the Mundugumor (New Guinea) males and females. Aggressive, belligerent behavior was common to both males and females, and both males and females were hostile to their children.

The Tschambuli tribesmen in New Guinea presented what could be regarded, by American standards, as a reversal of social roles. The women displayed more initiative and more businesslike manners than men.

Some of the so-called masculine and feminine traits are culturally imposed. The Tschambuli imposed certain behavioral patterns on their children, demanding aggressiveness in

boys and submissiveness in girls. Some American Indians
expected fearless behavior in boys. Little boys who failed to
conform and who displayed weakness and admitted fear or
pain were ostracized from the male gender and forced to join
the subservient female gender. They were treated like trans-
vestites, and forced to do women's work.

Some of the so-called feminine traits are culturally induced behavioral patterns (Mead, 1950) and some are direct
products of male wishes. In prehistorical times when children were the main labor force, having numerous children
was an economic necessity. Men who owned many child-
bearing women were economically prosperous and polygamy
was a sound economic device.

Some of the so-called feminine traits originated in the
socioeconomic structure of bygone times. A woman's task was
to produce babies and take care of them; a man's task was to
hunt, fish, fight, work, and provide food and protection.
Motherly love and care were praised as feminine traits; courage and cunning, as male traits. Women needed no initiative,
for their way of life was rather sedentary. While staying home,
they were expected to mind the hearth, cook meals, and keep
the house clean. Men were supposed to fight hostile neighbors
and beasts, be brave and aggressive. Men were expected to
fertilize several women; thus, they were expected to be sexually aggressive. Women were supposed to attract the male;
thus they were expected to be sweet, charming, and subservient. For millennia, women have been economically dependent on men. Women kept by men, whether in or outside
marriage, have received all the benefits as long as men cared
about them. Small wonder that a woman is taught "to lie to
men, to scheme, to be wiley. In speaking to them she wears
an artificial expression on her face; she is cautious, hypocrit-
ical, play-acting" (de Beauvoir, 1953, p. 259).

Apparently women have had no choice but to accept their passive, subservient role of charming girls, subservient wives, and caring mothers. From their earliest days, they were brainwashed and conditioned to accept their social role.

PENIS ENVY

There is no evidence for penis envy in earlier times when women seemingly accepted their subservient social position. In Freud's times, many little girls wished they were boys, for they believed that was the only way of escaping discrimination and subservience. Boys could go wherever they pleased, talk to whomever they wished, and choose the occupation they liked, but a girl was her father's slave until he transferred her to her future husband.

Freud did not invent penis envy, but discovered this phenomenon. It stands to reason that the more restrictions were imposed on girls, the more frequent was the wish to escape the yoke by a magic switching to the opposite sex. Some of my female patients dreamed about switching the railroad tracks.

Penis envy was never a general feeling common to all women at all times; certainly the Tschambuli or Arapesh women never had any reason for such an envy. Arapesh men and women shared household and child-rearing responsibilities, and the Tschambuli women were the dominant sex.

Freud's clinical observations of penis envy in women who were reared in an atmosphere of discrimination and subjugation must be interpreted in light of another hypothesis brought forward by Freud, namely, the tendency of the child to identify with the "strong aggressor." In patriarchal families, the father was the absolute ruler, and the male and female children were proud to identify with the father rather than the mother (Wolman, 1984).

In 20 years of clinical practice in this country, I have had a great many women patients. Going through my case reports, I arrived at the conclusion that penis envy was more frequent among the older generation of women, brought up in traditional father-controlled families with a clear male supremacy, than in the younger generation of women brought up in families with a tenuous or nonexistent father supremacy. Freud's observation of identification with the stronger parental figure seems to have been corroborated by my cases.

One must therefore interpret penis envy in girls not as an envy of their little brothers or playmates but rather as a wish for the possession of male freedom and power. Penis envy does not seem to be a general and universal element of female psychology, but should be perceived as the feminine protest against male domination. The penis as power symbol elicited well-understood feelings of envy.

Victor Hugo wrote that no power in the world can stop an idea when its time has come. The myth of passive femininity was challenged by hungry women who marched on Versailles at the onset of the French Revolution. Female factory workers joined the males in strikes and class struggle. Women began to demand equal rights, and the suffragist movement paved the road for the contemporary women's liberation movement.

Today, some women wish to be men, but some men wish to be women. Some of my male patients had dreams in which their wish to be a woman was clearly expressed. Female breasts appeared in the dreams as a cherished possession, and penises and breasts have often been confused.

My clinical experience makes me believe that neither men nor women can completely resolve their oedipal involvements, whether the positive ones (with the parent of the opposite sex) or the negative (with the parent of the same sex). Some residuum of the "first love" for the parent or the parent substitute seems to remain forever in almost all people.

The gradually increasing incidence of breast envy requires further study. At the present time, all that can be said is sociocultural speculation. It seems that many ideas, theories, and even empirical studies have been influenced by the sociocultural setting. For instance, it was a widely accepted belief that men are assertive and aggressive while women are compassionate and sympathetic. Today, several studies indicate that aggressiveness is not limited to one sex only (Bandura, 1973; Hamburg and Trudeau, 1984; Keith, 1984; Mednick and Christiansen, 1980; Valzelli, 1981).

In summary, the terms "masculine" and "feminine" are meaningless as long as they are indiscriminately applied. There are no "masculine" or "feminine" occupations; in France, Germany, and several other countries, men are teachers. In the Soviet Union, the majority of physicians are women. Men and women can be lawyers, mathematicians, elevator operators, mountain climbers, farmers, dentists, mailroom clerks, gynecologists, salespersons, psychiatrists, and so on. Sexual primary and secondary traits have precious little to do with one's occupation, intelligence, tenacity, moods, and so on. Some men (and some women) are more aggressive or more enterprising, or more anxious or more healthy, or more sick or more neurotic than other people, irrespective of their sex. The whole idea of male or female personality traits is a heritage from bygone times when men owned and controlled and programmed and brainwashed women (Williams, 1977).

FROM PROCREATION TO PLEASURE

Although the sexual drive is not an offshoot of the drive for survival, it is considerably influenced by the latter. For one thing, badly wounded and gravely ill people do not display much sexual craving, and no one thinks of sex when faced with mortal danger.

Moreover, sexual development is associated with the feeling of power. Children crave to become as big and strong as they believe the "grown-ups" are. But to be a grown-up means to become either a man or a woman, and quite early in life children make their choice. Usually the child identifies with the parent or parental substitute of the same sex.

This psychosexual identification is of utmost importance in developing one's self-image and self-esteem as a "real man," or a "real woman." Alfred Adler (1929) hypothesized a universal feminine feeling of inferiority, thus bringing to the extreme Freud's theory of penis envy. Most probably at the crossroads of the nineteenth and twentieth centuries, in the prudish, Victorian Vienna, many women felt inferior, but this phenomenon was far from being universal and had nothing to do with the alleged (sexual) organ inferiority. At all times and in all cultures a vast majority of children accept their body and its organs, and wish to grow up in their own gender. The growth of secondary sexual signs at puberty is viewed by most adolescents as proof of reaching adulthood and accepted with pride. Slow maturation often is a source of worry and concern.

With the beginning of active sexual life in adolescence or early adulthood sexual power plays a highly significant role in one's self-esteem, that is, estimate of one's power. In primitive societies men took pride in their ability to fertilize women and thus procreate the clan. Fertile women took pride in the number of children they could bring into the world, and the value of sexual prowess was measured by the number of children.

With the increase of population and apparent danger of overpopulation other aspects of sexuality come to the fore. The gradual change of the role of women and the new aspects of male–female relations have brought an increased emphasis on the ability to satisfy each other in sexual relations.

SEX AND LOVE

Sexual intercourse is practiced by all biological species that reproduce sexually. In a vast majority of cases sexual relations are void of any emotional factors; certainly one cannot ascribe affection to copulating insects. There is no doubt, however, that love originates in sexuality. Love could be best defined as a desire to take care of, to protect, and to give pleasure. Freud's concept of Eros combines the ideas of life and love, protection and pleasure. (Freud, 1949; Pribram and Gill, 1966; Wolman, 1984; Wolman and Money, 1980).

At a certain evolutionary level two types of love appear, namely, the sexual love between mating partners and the maternal love for the offspring.

The ethologist Konrad Lorenz described the continuous cooperation and mutual assistance between male and female cichlids, as follows:

> For the first time in the ascending ranks of the scale of living creatures, we see in these cichlids, a type of behavior which human beings consider highly moral; male and female remain in close connubial partnership even after reproduction is completed.... It is usually described as "marriage" when both partners together fence for the brood, though, for this purpose, no really

personal ties need exist between male and female; but in
cichlids they do exist. (1966, p. 36)

When Lorenz "swapped the wives" of the two male
cichlids, "the fish which had received the 'prettier' female"
was content with the exchange, but the one who received
the formerly rejected female in place of his wife attacked
her relentlessly. Lorenz was convinced that the fish noticed the difference (1966, p. 40). Some primitive human
beings would not notice; they practice sex on an instrumental level, seeking their own gratification only, and they obtain it with anyone. The other human being does not matter
to them, and human relations between two individuals are
reduced to copulation.

There is a clear connection between sexuality on one side
and the above-mentioned three types of social relations,
namely, the *instrumental* taking attitude, the *mutual* give-and-
take attitude, and the *vectorial* giving attitude, on the other.
The not-yet-born and the newborn infant's attitude is thor-
oughly instrumental; he must take in order to survive.
He may "love" his parents but he "loves" to be taken care
of by them. The infant's attitude is parasitic and his "love"
is exploitive.

It might be useful at this junction to repeat the definition
of love. Love is the desire to protect, to support, to defend,
and to satisfy needs. People can love in several different ways,
to a various degrees, and for a host of reasons. Some people
care for those who satisfy their needs. They do not want to
lose the givers. They do not want to give up a milk cow, an
egg-laying hen, or a workhorse. Owners "love" their property
and are ready to take care of and to defend it. This instrumental kind of "love" is typical of an infant. The infant loves
to take, and "loves" those who take care of him and as long
as they take care of him.

When a woman marries a man for his checkbook or when a man marries a woman because she can satisfy his sexual needs in addition to serving him as a cleaning maid and cook, this type of "love" is instrumental. Perhaps the term "love" does not agree with instrumental attitude for an instrumental attitude is basically self-love. Narcissistic psychopaths love themselves and use others. They are ready to protect those who allow themselves to be used and hate those who refuse to serve them.

The term "love" should be used only when people are willing to give, to protect, to care. Vectorial love represents the desire to give without expecting anything in return. Pregnancy is a case in point. The mother's organism serves the not-yet-born organism, supplies oxygen, food, and water and receives nothing in return.

VECTORIALISM

While parenthood offers the most natural outlet for vectorial love, it is not the only one. There are people who never have children and those who do, all let their children go at some point. Also, many people need additional outlets in addition to or instead of parenthood.

The need for a vectorial, giving-without-receiving pattern of relationship can be explained as follows. The less power one possesses, that is, the "poorer" one is, the greater is his need for supplies from without. Poor souls *must* be instrumental. As one grows stronger and has more to offer to others, he becomes capable of a give-and-take relationship. He may still be instrumental in certain areas, while in others he becomes mutual. A further increase in power leads to an overflow, and men with abundant energy need to discharge it. A milk cow must give away some of her milk, a creative artist seeks expression, and a man with a rich emotional life loves to love.

All this is vectorialism—giving without asking anything in return. One may invoke at this point Gesell's structure–function principle: When the structure is ready, the function begins (Gesell, 1928). When the child's bones and muscles are ready the child begins to walk. When his somatopsychic structure is ripe to start a new function, this new function begins.

No human being is capable of a complete and total vectorialism, for no human being is endowed with absolute power. All men are mortal and death is the inescapable limit to human power and pride.

There are, however, cases when the love for other, be it a person or an idea, may become stronger than the love for oneself. This type of a love, the Antigone principle (Wolman, 1965), applies more often to nonsexual love than to sexual love. A loving parent will give away the last piece of bread for his hungry child and, in mortal danger, he may sacrifice his own life to save the child.

One may vectorially love not only one's own children but all children and all those who need love and help. There are emotionally rich individuals capable of giving their abundant love to others. These individuals are inclined to act in a vectorial manner whenever the circumstances call for such an action. They display selfless love for others and act in a genuinely selfless manner. When charity is practiced for self-aggrandizement and publicity, it is instrumental. Charity becomes vectorial only when it aims for the well-being of its recipients. Self-sacrifice for one's religious beliefs and heroic deeds aimed at freedom for others are proofs of vectorial love.

Vectorial love may turn also toward nonhumans, such as inanimate objects and abstract concepts and ideas. People may sacrifice their lives for objects of arts, scientific convictions, and religious beliefs. Giordano Bruno, the early Christians in times of the Roman persecutions, and the Jews throughout the ages have shown the willingness to lose their lives for what they believed in.

There is one type of vectorial love that does not impoverish the giver: Creative work does not make one poor. The origin of creativity is procreation. The man who fertilizes a woman in the embrace of love does not impoverish himself nor does the beloved woman. Giving birth does not make a woman less of what she was.

Sublimated libido can be invested in creative, scientific, or artistic work without any loss to oneself. Great poets, painters, and composers have cathected their desexualized libido in their work, and the more they created the greater was their talent to create more.

Society perpetuates itself not only in a biological sense but also in a sociocultural sense. Whatever people have created, future generations may continue, carry on, and enjoy. Great works of art and science are not transmitted through genes but through books, schools, and other media of communication. Thus giving new ideas, creating works of art and science, and giving to humanity are acts of survival. Procreation is the physical survival of humanity. Creation of cultural values is the spiritual, symbolic, and everlasting survival of humanity. Procreation preserves the human race as a collective biological organism. Cultural creativity preserves humanity on its road above biology. It is the process of *becoming*, becoming less animalistic and more human.

It is irrelevant whether Socrates and Homer, Ovid and Virgil, Thomas Aquinas and Maimonides, Da Vinci and Michael Angelo, Mozart and Chopin had children, and whether their biological children continued the work of their fathers. Great geniuses are the fathers of us all. All of us who read and listen, who think and admire art and music are their children. They live in us and through us. Spinoza and Kant, Shakespeare and Tolstoy, Bartok and Bernstein, Modigliani and Picasso are the heirs of the great creators of the past, and in the future, creative men and women will continue the great heritage and perpetuate human survival. Mozart and Da Vinci and Shakespeare as biological organisms do not exist any longer, but their creative works live in us.

But the creative act itself is a source of self-fulfillment and self-enrichment irrespective of its future impact. Creative work is an evolvement of inner potentialities. It is a process of growth and ascension of new and higher levels. It is an act of *becoming*.

A rosebush that blossomed and the cherry tree that bore fruit fulfilled their inner potentialities irrespective of how many people were pleased with the fragrance of roses and the taste of cherries. But the rosebush that did not blossom and the cherry tree that did not bear fruit have not become bigger, stronger, and better developed than the rosebush that gave hundreds of roses and the cherry tree that produced thousands of cherries. A poet who never wrote, a painter who never painted, a composer who never composed a melody were underachievers who led an underdeveloped, unfulfilled, wasted life.

MUTUALITY IN SEX

No human being can forever give without receiving anything in return. Adult sexuality is a give-and-take process.

Adult sexual intercourse is an expression of mutual attraction, affection, and tenderness. No one wants to hurt his partner in lovemaking, unless he is a pathological rapist or sadist. Sexual foreplay in normal adults is not a tug-of-war, but sweet talk, flattery, affectionate hugging, kissing, and petting. To be forceful does not mean to be hostile; one does not hug his girlfriend or wife to hurt her. Insertion and actual intercourse with a willing partner do not require aggression or violence. Hostility and violence elicit opposition to intimacy, and quarreling couples usually become sexually estranged. Violence during intercourse inflicts pain, and unless the partner is a masochist, the sensual pleasure is destroyed.

Adult sexuality is the prototype of mutual relations. Normal adults enjoy sexual relations as a sensual pleasure both for themselves and for their partner. It is a give-and-take relationship. One wants to give to his or her partner all the gratification, expecting that the partner is wishing the same. One enjoys receiving gratification and enjoys giving it to one for whom one cares. Sensual pleasure becomes enhanced by affection and friendliness (Wolman and Money, 1980).

Sexuality in normal adults transcends its physiological foundations, and the choice of a sexual partner is rarely purely physical. People are not attracted to each other's sexual organs, but to an overall impression they make. Physical appearance, pleasant manners, color of eyes and hair, smile, timbre of voice, self-assuredness, promise of fulfillment, kindness, and several other behavioral patterns serve as cues. Were physiology the sole determinant of sexual choice, there would be very little to say about it, for all men and women have appropriate sexual organs.

The choice of a partner is based upon a variety of nonsexual factors. One is attracted to a girl before one sleeps with her; and more lasting choices are based on mutual understanding, kindness, and affection rather than on physiology. Often factors not related to sexuality determine marital choice. Men and women may love each other and live happily together even though they have married for monetary or status reasons, or when intellectual affinity or practical considerations brought them together. The physiological aspect is an indisputable, but is not the sole determinant of adult sexuality. Genital organs are an indisputable element of adult sexuality, but the choice of a partner, the nature, and longevity of the relationship usually depend on mutual understanding, friendly disposition of the partners, cultural compatibility, and their interaction in daily life (Wolman and Stricker, 1983).

Mature adult sexual choice is monogamous and tends to be lasting. Obviously, one cannot have sexual intercourse with more than one person at the same time. If sexual relations and other aspects of being together are gratifying, one does not look for a change. One seeks change when the present situation is unpleasant, but even then one does not look for numbers, but for one satisfactory and lasting relationship (Wolman and Money, 1980).

SOCIOCULTURAL DETERMINANTS

At all times and in all societies, the nature of sexual relations was regulated by social norms. In many instances religion determined the rights and wrongs in male–female relations. Even today the Catholic religion does not approve of divorce and abortion. Most societies restrain sexual freedom, forbid incest, rape, and sex with minors, and several societies forbid adultery, prostitution, and homosexuality.

Every society tries to regulate sexual relations in accordance with the prevailing beliefs and norms. Sometimes sex is controlled by law, and sometimes public opinion is the main regulating force. There is, however, no social system totally oblivious of the fact that sex involves more than one person, and as such it represents a highly important avenue of interindividual relations that cannot be totally free. For one

thing, marriage and family are highly important social, cultural, and economic institutions, and no society can let them
become too wayward.

The sexual urge has always been a natural urge, just as
hunger and the need for protection from enemies, but neither
sex nor hostility can be dealt with outside a broader context
of social interaction. Therefore, psychology of sexuality must
not be analyzed outside the fundamental drive for survival.

This shift of emphasis from Eros, libido, and sexuality in
the direction of survival and adjustment to life follow, to a
certain extent, the ideas of Hartmann, Kardiner, and Erikson,
but one may reinterpret several aspects of psychosexual development and sexual behavior in the light of the fundamental
lust for life drive. In the phylogenetic development of nature,
the fight for survival was the earliest and most fundamental
driving force, while sexual procreation appeared much later
in the process of evolution. With exceedingly rare exceptions,
the urge to live is always more powerful than the urge to love,
and sexual behavior is greatly influenced by the more basic
needs related to survival.

Marriage and family are institutions primarily geared to
sexual relations and child rearing, but economic factors are of
utmost importance in marital contracts. Economic aspects of
marital life have determined the fate and structure of the
various types of family organization.

In primitive societies power was in numbers. The more
warriors, the more power, and the better chance to defend
own territory and to grab territories belonging to other groups
or tribes. The more men, the better chance for its survival.

Sex has been the main factor in propagation of the species,
the herd, the tribe. The more sex, the better chances for group
survival. In many primitive societies the phallus has become
the symbol of power and the guardian of group survival.

Since the inception of mankind human beings have been proud of their ability to produce children. Practically all primitive religions worshipped masculine and feminine fertility, and Osiris, Baal, Zeus, Kibola, and Gea are names of gods–fathers and goddesses–mothers. Reproduction serves the function of preservation of the species, and in ancient times lack of fertility represented a threat to the survival of the society.

Primitive economies were based primarily on the availability of labor force; thus families with many children were better off than those who had only few children. Production of children was one of the most important aspects of the economy, and polygamy was the choice method. Child-bearing women were held in high esteem, and childless ones were often sent back to their parents' homes. At the time of Roman Empire and its conquests, which brought mass slavery, the size of the family had declined and homosexuality had become a widespread phenomenon.

SEX AND THE ABUSE OF POWER

Sex in human beings can be practiced on the lowest and the highest evolutionary level. The fact that several curse words are related to sex and numerous derogatory expressions denote sexual organs and performance bear witness to the ambivalent feelings people have about sex. An inadequate, stupid man is described in vulgar terms identifying him as the male sexual organ; parallel expressions describe stupid women.

Sex is one of the fundamental physiological needs, but it is also associated with friendliness, affection, and a feeling of security. People boast with material achievements for they provide for food, clothing, and shelter, and many men and women derive a great deal of self-esteem from their sexual prowess.

Men often boast about their sexual potency; it is their ability to satisfy women. Beginners brag about their achievements, sexual and others. Erection is a source of pleasure and pride in the phallic stage. Most men retain some show-off tendencies. Arab males swear on mustaches, a symbol of masculinity in their culture. Ancient Romans put all lofty and noble traits together under the name *virtus,* coined from the Latin word *vir,* which means "man." In colloquial English, to "talk man to man" is believed to be more dignified or truthful or important than to talk to a woman.

Sexual behavior has been for millennia a sign and symbol of power. Strong men were believed to be able to perform well sexually, make many women pregnant, and have a great deal of children. In some primitive tribes, the number of children was indicative of the manly power of the father.

Sex represents a great many symbolic indicators of the feeling of power. In some higher mammals, males chase after females and coerce them, not really against their will but to some extent with a great deal of game playing, displaying their power. Some mammals compete for females, the big walrus, who can control a big harem, probably feels stronger than those who are unable to have as many females, or no females at all. For a great many years, men had to buy females or conquer them. In the Old Testament, the story is told about the forefathers who had to work for many years before they were able to earn enough income to pay off the price of the females. Ancient Romans raped the Sabine women. Women were an object to be taken, conquered, bought, and sold; thus a strong man was a man who could get as many women as possible. Then he would sleep with them, and make them pregnant. In our times, some men are boastful about their success with women, ignoring the fact that contemporary women neither wear chastity belts nor are they impenetrable fortresses. Some men who have nothing else to be proud of tend to boast about their sexual powers. Impotent or self-conscious men boast about their conquests, and insecure women who doubt their femininity practice promiscuity as if this was the only way of proving their femininity (Williams, 1977; Wolman and Money, 1980).

Even today, adolescents and immature adults boast about their sexual achievements as if sleeping with a woman was something unusual and a unique sign of masculine power. So many people believe that sexual performance is a sign of power, and many men play the role of Don Juan, feeling that having a great many women is a sign of heroic achievement. Actually Don Juan is a symbol of a man who is afraid of women, afraid of making commitments to one woman, and therefore runs from one woman to another. He does not chase after them, but he escapes them. The need of weak individuals to prove how great they are makes men into Don Juans and women promiscuous. People who doubt their power or their achievement or their skill show off more than those who are self-confident.

Hostile behavior has been often related to the male sex hormone (Keith, 1984; Valzelli, 1981; Wolman and Money, 1980). Removal of the hormone caused a reduction in both sexual and aggressive behavior. However, Bevan, Daves, and Levy (1960) have shown that the most belligerent animals were those who have had successful fighting experience in the past, irrespective of their possession or loss of sexual organs.

Several authors viewed sexual rivalry among males as the main reason for hostility. However, Bovet described herds of cattle in Switzerland with a highly aggressive female as the head (Mead, 1950). Apparently nature is all but uniform, and biology can offer empirical support for practically any psychological hypothesis. The only thing one may say is that stronger animals, as a rule, display more intraspecific aggression than weaker ones. Strong males are usually more overtly aggressive than weak females; stronger creatures are usually more offensive, weaker ones more defensive.

Observations in wards of mental hospitals do not support the hypothesis of females being less hostile than males, and counting the number of physical fights in male and female wards or the number of children's fights in schools could not offer convincing proof either.

Because women are physically weaker than men, and they are less prone toward and less trained to use physical force. Our society frowns on physical hostility in women, but even a casual observer can easily notice that women compensate very well for their physical inferiority, and hostile behavior is just as frequent among them as among men. Unfair judgment, malicious gossip, intentional hurting of feelings, slander, and insult are at least as frequent among women in girls' schools, offices, factories, laboratories, and stores as they are among men in comparable situations. The alleged feminine kindness is a myth. The Nazi women organized in *Bund Deutscher Mädels* were as antihuman, heartless, and cruel as their male counterparts. The notorious Ilse Koch who made lampshades out of human skin had scores of feminine associates who actively participated in looting and murder. Nazi women were less active in the actual act of murder than were the men for the sole reason that women are physically weaker than men. In prejudice, hate, incitement to violence, and malice the role of females is indisputable.

The belief in feminine kindness and angellike behavior is a part of man's mother idolatry. Adoration of mother is typical for both male and female infants. Infants "love" the "good" mother who satisfies their wishes but they hate the same mother when she refuses to meet their demands. Ambivalent feelings toward powerful protectors are an inevitable product of dependence, and they often carry the seeds of rebellion against being weak and dependent. Poor relatives often resent their wealthy supporters.

The ambivalent feeling toward the mother is shared by little boys and little girls, and this attitude has been perpetuated throughout generations taking on various forms and shapes. Rarely if ever can a woman resolve completely her antimother feelings. In Freud's times, it was acceptable for young women to displace hatred onto their mothers-in-law. Freud interpreted this phenomenon as a residue of the castration complex; be it as he wrote, the symbolic loss of a penis represented a loss of power and of the privileged male status.

The boys' ambivalent feelings toward the mother has been often channeled into the "macho" complex. Even the most cowardly and ineffectual men can play the role of a strong man and discharge brute force toward someone weaker than themselves. Women were the choice target, and the male-controlled public opinion favored the "masculine assertion" toward women and children.

The possession of a penis has given the men an additional tool used for the humiliation of women and for self-aggrandizement. The sexual act as such is neither beautiful nor ugly and like almost everything else in human life, it can be practiced in a most lofty and most base manner. However, the allegedly aggressive and domineering sexual insertion was often represented as an act of debasement of women.

The ambivalent male attitude toward women has been immortalized in poetry and in obscenity. Poets sang songs of the beautiful godlike creatures they admired and desired, while less sophisticated men used colorful terms to denote their disrespect for whatever one can do with women. This polarization has been well expressed in the adoration of the mother image and the malicious persecution of women accused of witchcraft (Williams, 1977).

EMANCIPATION OF WOMEN

Errors die hard and the owl of wisdom is a notorious latecomer. The demand for equal rights for women came one century later than it was due. The emancipation of women was started by men themselves for a less than noble reason: men needed women to work for them.

The Industrial Revolution with its insatiable need for working hands pulled thousands of women away from the hearth and crib. The decline of the feudal system and the rapidly diminished role played by agriculture forced masses of women into the open labor markets of the budding capitalist economy.

Women's participation in the production and distribution of goods has irrevocably changed their psychosocial roles. The privileged and respected role of provider, which was the backbone of the traditional male-dominated family structure, began to crack and presently it is heading toward a hitherto unknown crisis.

The erosion of the traditional male–female relationship started first in the lowest and then in the highest social classes. The middle classes have been notoriously the bulwark of conservatism.

The present-day family constellation deprived the father of his authority but it did not replace it by any other authority. One cannot help wondering what is going to happen in our times to the Oedipus complex, latency period, and the whole area of male–female relationships. Modern women have destroyed the myth of their intellectual inferiority and denied, *in vivo*, the assumption of their alleged angel or witch personality (Wolman and Stricker, 1983).

Not all men love women, nor do all men hate them, nor does the one attitude exclude the other. There has been a good deal of speculation and little factual knowledge concerning the characteristics of the two sexes and their interaction, though this area of behavior is secondary in importance to breadwinning behavior only. From the inception of sexual reproduction, that is, since the times when females began to bear children, the child–mother relationship has been the first social and emotional experience in everyone's life. The first prenatal impressions are the intrauterine ones; the first serious shock of separation is birth; the first sensations of hunger, thirst, satiation, comfort, warmth, and security are experienced by the infant in the relationship with his mother or maternal substitute.

The subservient and submissive role of women is rapidly coming to an end. The abuse of physical strength in male–female relationship is not related to sexuality as such but to human belligerence to be described below.

HOSTILE BEHAVIOR

A search for the origins of life-promoting and life-destroying behavior may proceed in the direction of phylogenesis, ontogenesis, or both. Both phylogenetic and ontogenetic studies bear unmistakable evidence to the fact that all creatures eat and reproduce. Higher animals apparently get excited about food and sex, but sex is not as universal a trait as is the intake of food. All living organisms take in food, but sex started much later in the process of evolution. Let us therefore begin our discussion with the behavior patterns related to the survival of the individual, such as eating and defenses against being eaten (Bandura, 1973; Hamburg and Trudeau, 1981).

Eating, fighting, destructiveness, aggression, murder, and war are common occurrences in animal and human life. Let us call all behavior that aims at hurting, harming, damaging, and eventually destroying another organism "hostility." The term hostility or hostile behavior will be used consistently in the following pages. I suggest that we abandon the ambiguous terms "aggressive" and "aggressiveness," for to be aggressive may also mean to be resourceful, forceful, energetic, and bold with or without harm to others.

Although the term hostility implies destructive action of one or more individuals, hostility may also turn inward in self-defeating, self-damaging, and suicidal acts.

Hostility may also be aimed at inanimate nature and verbal and nonverbal symbols, whenever these objects or symbols represent or stand for organisms. One may willfully destroy an enemy's property thus hurting the enemy; one may burn books, flags, and other objects that symbolize the enemy, his beliefs, and ways of life.

A distinction between hostile actions and hostile feelings or hate is necessary. Hostility is the name for overt behavior that aims at damage or complete destruction. Hate is not necessarily part of overt behavior. A prisoner of war hates his captors, yet he does not hurt them.

While hostile behavior is observable, hate is not always observable, yet it is an empirical fact, it takes place, and can be assessed. It is a part of behavior, sometimes overt, sometimes covert.

Animals fight not to kill but to survive. In order to eat, they must kill and they do. Whenever someone wants to eat them, they fight to kill—to kill the enemy so that they can survive. When someone else has what they need, whether it be food, water, a cave to hide in, a female, a treasury, a place under the sun, or natural resources, they fight with him to get what they need. Whoever fights, fights a real fight and not a "ritualistic" one. Animals and men fight to kill in order to get what they want. When the enemy surrenders or runs away and the victor gets the spoil, the victor will usually not pursue further unless he is afraid that the victim may come back. In such a case it is safest to kill the dangerous enemy.

Some students of hostile behavior seem to be surprised that hostility can occur independent of eating. Except for the relationship of predator to prey, animals rarely destroy members of other species. Overt fighting to kill rarely occurs in vertebrates, and probably never occurs in mammals living under natural conditions.

Man appears to be an exception. Human belligerence resulted in the death of 59,000,000 human beings from wars and persecution between the years 1820 and 1945. Lorenz wrote:

> There are very few animals which, even when threatened with starvation, will attack an equal sized animal of their own species with the intention of devouring it. I only know this to be definitely true of rats and a few related rodents.... But Dytiscus larvae devour animals of their own breed and size, even when other nourishment is at hand, and that is done, as far as I know, by no other animal. (1966, p. 21).

In primates and in the human race, cannibalism is an exception rather than the rule. Men do not kill men to eat them, but kill for more or less the same reasons as other animals do. They fight not for the sake of fighting but for the sake of winning (Hamburg and Trudeau, 1981).

Most mammals fight in the mating process. As a rule, they usually do not fight to the death because the weaker male runs away. The desire to survive apparently rates higher than the sex urge. The victor has no reason to kill the competitor; all he wants is the female, and once he has won, there is no need to kill the loser. While the fight goes on, it is not "ritualized" or gentle. It is a real fight with teeth and claws, and severe wounds are inflicted. Death is not the goal; it is the means toward survival or toward the satisfaction of a need.

Human beings are the only species always ready to fight big wars on battlefields and little wars when they convert the family dining tables into battlefields. They kill one another for distant oil wells, for nearby coal mines, for political freedom, for political domination, for the King and Honor, for moral principles or against them, for religious beliefs in the name of the God of Mercy or against disbelievers, for freedom of speech or against those who dare to question, and even for strategic positions that would enable them to wage future wars. Some people are eager to practice violence in the name of peace. Hungry lions roar; belligerent human beings often profess peace and wage a war against those who stand in their way. Since it is impossible to find two individuals who always agree with one another, physical and verbal fights have continued unabated since the earliest days of mankind.

There is no conclusive evidence regarding ethnic inclinations to wage war. Historians have registered about 2,600 battles among European nations in the years 1480–1940. During this period Russia's and Prussia's warlike participation was continuously on the increase, while Holland, Spain, and the Scandinavian nations have shown a decrease in warfare. Austria, England, France, and Turkey did not display much change in their warlike attitudes during the entire period.

Wars have several varied causes. It would be rather a gross distortion of truth to assume that all wars have been imperialistic or patriotic or motivated by a simple acting out of hostile impulses. There have been aggressive and defensive wars as well wars fought for conquest, oil wells, ideological reasons, hurt pride, false ambitions, and dire necessity to defend oneself.

Many aggressive wars, such as the continuous strife between ancient Egypt and the Mesopotamian kings of Assyria and Babylonia, were largely preventive wars aimed at the destruction of a threatening enemy. Want and fear of enemies are apparently quite frequent causes of wars. In either case, survival is a true or imaginary or fabricated reason most often used as an excuse for wars, and paranoia is one of the most common traits of individuals and groups.

Animals fight *against* each other for food, but people could work *together* instead of fighting. There is a reasonably good chance for peaceful cooperation in work and civilization starts when people turn swords into plowshares. Ferocious animals fight for survival with teeth and claws, but civilized men can *produce* whatever they need. Group living in civilized societies does not prevent intragroup strife, but it facilitates cooperation in producing goods and services that everyone needs.

Reduction of fear reduces hostile feelings. People do not hate butterflies, doves, kittens, and infants, but they hate poisonous snakes, biting rats, wolves, and gangsters. Fear is reduced when one is strong enough to defend oneself or when there is sufficient outside protection.

Fear motivates individuals and nations to arm to teeth, ready to fight enemies. *Si vis pacem, para bellum* (if you want peace, prepare for war), the ancient Romans used to say. "Armed peace," "balance of power," and "armament race" are three synonymous concepts of modern times. Friendly people are prone to solve their differences in an amicable way, but even friendship does not prevent conflicts of interests. Whenever people wish something and cannot get it, they may feel like fighting for it.

The theory that frustration leads to aggression tells the obvious and offers no solution to the problem. Frustration calls forth an aggressive desire to overcome it. In most cases hostility is directed toward the true or imaginary source of frustration. In many cases hostile feelings and behavior are displaced in scapegoating and in others they turn inward, against oneself.

Obviously, if all human wishes were fulfilled, there would be no reason for hostile behavior. But such utopian, perfect, ideal state of affairs is impossible. Certainly, social and political systems can be improved, and more food and more security for all could be provided. But no social system can remove human desires, whims, ambitions, likes, and dislikes, and no social order can prevent interindividual tensions. Even identical twins may clash and the most loving husband and wife may disagree and frustrate each other.

In a large society conflicts of interest are inevitable. Conflicts of interest are likely to occur between labor and management, buyers and salesmen, and any other group or groups of people. No society, as perfect as it may be, can abolish conflict once and for all.

The question is whether fighting and war could be prevented. The first step is to reduce the apparent reason for fighting, such as want and fear. No one can tell whether these two factors and especially the latter could be ever completely removed. A powerful supreme body of justice, such as proposed by Freud, could be of great help if it ever came into being.

However, the most important and decisive step would be a voluntary renunciation of violence in human relations.

Are people capable of a voluntary renunciation of violence? Chapter 5 will deal with personality development and morality.

5

Child Development

THE TWO PERSPECTIVES

Child development must be viewed in a dual perspective of natural, biologically determined developmental phases on the one hand and social and cultural factors related to the child's interaction with his family and other individuals on the other. These two sets of factors are closely interrelated, for the way a child goes through the natural developmental phases hypothesized by Freud, Gesell, or Piaget greatly depends on the child's environment, which may facilitate or hamper the child's growth and development.

Two concepts of developmental phases must be critically examined from a sociocultural perspective. Consider insects. Their developmental phases are clearly determined in a sequence of egg, larva, cocoon, and adult insect. Hardly any insect remains "fixated" in one of the early phases and hardly if ever could an insect become an "immature adult." Short of a major physical impairment, all insects follow developmental phases common to a particular biological species.

A similar but more flexible statement could be applied to higher biological species. Consider mammals. All of them are sexually reproduced and all of them live, for a while, an intrauterine, prenatal life. None of them at birth is ready to procure food and shelter for himself, and usually they require a considerable period of parental care before they reach maturity and are really on their own.

The higher the species, the longer is the road from birth to maturity. Human neonates compare unfavorably with other mammals. They are, as it were, born prematurely, totally unable to survive unless taken care of. Human infants need a long time before they attain any degree of self-sufficiency.

This period of transition from infancy to adulthood becomes prolonged in modern societies. Primitive tribes practiced puberty rites that celebrated a quick transition. The rites are sort of a test of adulthood, and the young who passed them are admitted to the community of adults. As an adult, one is expected to earn a living, to marry, and to support a family. Physical maturity is expected to coincide with sociocultural maturity and, accordingly, social status is changed from a child to an adult. In the ancient Jewish tradition, the Bar Mitzvah ceremony signaled the beginning of *responsibility.* Until the age of 13, the boy's sins were blamed on his father, but from this age on the boy was held responsible for his actions.

The transition from childhood to adulthood is not an easy task in any society but the complexity of modern societies creates additional difficulties for the young. The age of physical maturation has not changed much in the course of millennia, but the concept of psychosocial maturity has undergone substantial changes.

Physical and sexual maturity is attained at the age of 15 to 18 for boys, 13 to 16 for girls, but boys and girls in their teens are unable to support themselves nor are they capable of assuming responsibility for family relationships. A technological society has no use for juvenile shepherds and hunters, and the modern economic system is based on skilled labor and highly qualified managerial and professional cadres. A grade school dropout can hardly earn a living in our society, and there are fewer and fewer job opportunities for unskilled labor. Prolonged schooling is needed for economic adjustment and adequate psychocultural maturity is a prerequisite for an adult participation in modern societies. Such a social–economic–cultural maturity requires a high level of psychological development, which can hardly be attained in the teens (Maccoby, 1984).

The concept of biological developmental phases cannot be rigidly applied at all times to all societies. The changing sociocultural climate requires revision of developmental concepts and their adjustment to the new conditions. Erikson (1963) suggested one of the possible modifications of Freud's developmental stages. The following will describe another modification.

NATURE–NURTURE

A newborn child comes to the world with a certain biochemical endowment. Biological factors hardly, if ever, change unless a particular child is exposed to atomic radiation or other chemical or physical factors. All children, with the rare exception of artificial insemination, are born of their mother's egg fertilized by their father's sperm, and a considerable part of their life journey is determined by the chromosomes and genes they received. Genetic factors will determine their physical appearance, and to a great extent their physical and mental health, their temperament, intellectual abilities, and even the speed of their development. There is ample evidence that intelligence, special abilities, and certain temperamental traits are carried by genes and thus form the basis for future development (Fuller & Simmel, 1983; Vandenberg & Vogler, 1985). Future development, however, is not a simple evolution of inherited traits but a series of interactional processes with one's physical and social environment. Even the healthiest seed will not grow and become a beautiful tree if it is kept in acid or freezing temperatures. The innate physical, chemical, and psychological dispositions may or may not come into fruition depending on environmental factors. The rapid development in neurochemical research (Filskov and Boll, 1981; Harmony, 1984) does not allow the view of human behavior as a purely psychogenic phenomenon. The sociocultural environment is no longer conducive to viewing behavior in a framework of stimulus–response or psychoanalytic constructs, as some human actions are influenced by a great many factors, starting with the genes (Vandenberg and Vogler, 1985).

The intrauterine life represents another set of determinants to account for. The physical and mental state of the mother can greatly influence the future development of the child. The mother's diet and emotional state and her intake of alcohol and drugs may foster or play havoc with the child's future mental health (Stechler and Halton, 1982).

All of these factors, however, are not the sole determinants of a child's development, and even innate constitutional shortcomings or defects can be totally or partially remedied by postnatal care.

It is, therefore, as naive to assume that one's physicochemical makeup dooms one to a certain pattern of living as it is to ignore the fact that they do have a powerful impact on a child's development, personality formation, and daily behavior. The following will describe the sociopsychological factors with the understanding that no matter how important they are, they are not the sole determinant of human behavior.

The basic elements of personality are determined by genes. Future physicochemical and psychosocial influences can exercise significant impact. They can help or harm the genetic predispositions, but a tree does not grow without a seed and personality development greatly depends on genetic background.

DEVELOPMENTAL PROCESSES

The entire process of development evolves according to the law of *negative acceleration.* Negative acceleration means a sequence of decreased increments. The child's progress, whether of physical height or intellectual development, gradually slows down. The developmental process has an immanent, built-in goal which is maturity. The progress toward the goal is rapid in prenatal and early life and it becomes slower and slower toward the end of the developmental process.

While the physical goal of maturity includes several clearly definable areas such as anatomy and physiology of the human organism, the concept of psychological maturity hinges on several factors of development and learning related to interaction with one's social environment.

There is an apparent gulf between physical and sociocultural maturity. People reach their full height and full development of anatomical structure and physiological functions in late adolescence. Their mental development takes usually much longer and it reaches maturity in postadolescent years, in adulthood. Adult, mature individuals do not "grow" any longer but they do *learn.* The learning process may continue until one's last breath.

The fact of continuous learning contradicts earlier hypotheses that implied that most aspects of personality structure are shaped in childhood. Apparently, in accordance with

Gesell's (1928) structure–function principle, certain periods are best suited for certain types of learning. For example, ballet dancing, violin playing, and certain other talents must be trained in childhood; if missed, they cannot be recaptured in later life. But a gifted person can start painting practically at any time in life.

As a rule, the older one is, the more difficult to condition new behavioral patterns and uncondition the old ones. But difficult as it may be, it is not impossible. The cathectic processes of love (libido) and hate (destrudo) continue uninterrupted throughout one's life, and new likes and dislikes come and go as long as one is alive, and certain aspects of personality can undergo changes even late in life.

The changes in conditioning and cathexes are caused by *interaction* with other people. Changes in interindividual libido and destrudo cathexes inevitably cause changes in the intraindividual balance of cathexes, that is, personality changes. An older person may feel isolated, which increases self-hatred and resentment against others. A significant personality change can take place when an active, busy, self-assured man is forced to retire and suddenly feels useless, helpless, and lonely. The bitterness is in some cases a product of hardening of the arteries, but in many cases it may be an artifact of discrimination against old age (Kahana, 1982).

I have treated men and women of various ages, some of them young and some old. I cannot say that older people have always been more difficult patients than the young ones. Some elderly people displayed mental alertness and willingness to change, and they underwent considerable personality changes in the process of psychotherapy.

Psychotherapy is a *field process,* just as any other interactional relationship. The relative balance of power of interacting people determines the degree of influence one can exercise. The same principle applies to all human relations, and especially to the child–parent interaction, where the parents wield considerable influence on the child's behavior and development.

PARENTS AND CHILDREN

There are two main reasons why children are less capable than adults of coping with their environment. Children are physically weaker and smaller, less experienced, and less wise than adults and therefore less capable of making rational decisions and implementing them. The younger they are, the less power they have, and they are less capable of sustaining themselves and conducting a successful struggle for survival. The second reason is their dependence, that is, the need to be accepted by others. Children's needs for support and allies is much greater than those of adults. Small children could not survive unless an adult takes care of them and supplies them with food, water, shelter, and protection against potential dangers. The dependence on outside support makes children fear rejection and abandonment (Wolman and Stricker, 1983).

In addition to these two main reasons, children have no say in choosing their environment and influencing their opportunities. Adults have some degree of mobility: they can change jobs, places of residence, marital relations, religion, business association, political affiliation, and so on, but children are born to and brought up by people they did not choose, and they are, indeed, the captive audience in their parents' homes.

Excluding major catastrophes such as earthquakes, wars, and economic upheavals, adults can live in a certain neighborhood, practice a certain occupation, develop friendly relations with business associates and relatives, and establish structured daily routines. Children do not have these options. Children may feel uprooted whenever their parents decide to change their place of residence, their family relationships, or any other social contacts.

Children have little power of their own, and their parents have all the power to promote or destroy their mental health. A self-confident person reacts to a danger with mobilization of his resources, but rejection, isolation, and abandonment adversely affect a child who has little self-confidence and practically no self-reliance.

Traumatized, hurt, and anxious children may regress to an earlier phase of development where they might feel better protected and more secure. A kindergarten-age child may regress to baby talk and a school age child may become a bed wetter.

Mature adults first count on themselves, and then on their friends, relatives, and others. Children must count first on others, on the loving and protecting parents or parental substitutes. Adults' security depends on power first and acceptance second; children's security depends on acceptance by others first and their own power next. Power has been defined as the ability to satisfy needs and survival is all encompassing and universal. Acceptance has been defined as the willingness to do so, that is, to satisfy the needs of other people, by helping and protecting them.

Every child must receive enough protection to enable him to function as a child. A child has the right to be a child, and as such he needs parental protection that gives him the feeling of security based on being accepted by his strong and friendly parents. The presence of loving parents or parental substitutes is necessary for his mental health and his development into a well-adjusted adult. A child needs cathecting supplies of parental libido in order to develop his own intraindividual balance of cathexes. Children need help in the process of growing up and reaching maturity. They must grow stronger and wiser and develop a realistic estimate of their physical and mental resources. They need help and encouragement in the natural process of shifting from a dependence on others toward a growing self-reliance (Wolman, 1982).

Mentally healthy individuals are realistic, and their perception of the world is pretty close to what the world is. They are capable of distinguishing wish from reality, and whenever they err, they test again and rectify their findings. The picture they have of themselves and others closely corresponds to the truth.

Children gradually develop the ability for reality testing. Children learn and mature gradually, and every child has his own biologically determined speed of maturational and innate ability to learn and profit from experience.

DEVELOPMENTAL PHASES

People are born *anomous*. They know of no restraint, no concern, no consideration for anyone. The intrauterine life is parasitic: the zygote–embryo–fetus is all out for itself and grabs whatever it can. Mother's body is self-sacrificing: whatever it possesses, it is ready to give to feed and to protect the not-yet-born child.

Birth changes little in the parasitic attitude. The newborn must use his or her own respiratory system, but the parasitic-dependent attitude continues. The infant wants what he wants and follows his instant stimuli and impulses. He operates on the principle of immediate gratification of needs called by Freud *Lustprinzip* (erroneously translated as the pleasure principle). Infants are anomous, that is amoral and limitlessly selfish.

The next phase starts with restraints imposed from without. Fear of retaliation and punishment is the first though preciously small step. The earliest restraints are based on fear; thus the earliest phase of primitive development should be called *phobonomous*. With the development of a rudimentary awareness of potential consequences, the child's selfishness faces restraints. He learns to obey because he fears. Fear is not morality, but primitive people and toddlers must be restrained from without. This restraint breaks the ground for a new phase of personality development.

As the child becomes aware of parental love and care, he appreciates what he gets and begins to reciprocate. His "love" is quite selfish, that is, instrumental, for he loves only those who love him. He wishes to protect them, for he needs their protection. The child needs parental love and fears he may lose it; thus his attitude toward the parents is a combination of love and fear. The child willingly and fearfully accepts parental rules and prohibitions, and gradually absorbs these rules and perceives them as if they were his own. He identifies with the parents or parental substitutes and incorporates their prohibitions and norms. He learns to blame himself for occasional disobedience and develops guilt feelings whenever he violates parental rules. His behavior is *heteronomous* for he willingly obeys norms instituted by others whom he perceives as loving and powerful authority figures. In Freud's personality model this self-regulatory agency was called superego.

Human personality does not reach its full development with childhood acceptance of parental rules and the formation of the superego. Preadolescents and adolescents develop close interpersonal relations with their peers and form groups, cliques, and gangs. Quite often these new social relations displace the child–parent attachments, and the rules of peer society become the ultimate source of behavior. The individual's willful identification with the peer group to which he chooses to belong becomes the guiding principle in his life for years to come, and often his loyalty goes on until the end of his life. This mutual acceptance of social norms, whether of a certain religious denomination, racial or ethnic group, or political party, leads to the formation of a new part of one's personality, which I would call the *we-ego*, and this group-identification period I shall call *socionomous*.

Most people do not go beyond the socionomy and acceptance of the norms prevailing in their particular group, clan subculture, or larger social segments. Most people follow certain binding rules of their particular group. They are "brothers" and "sisters" who abide by principles within their brotherhood and sisterhood.

The ultimate development goes beyond socionomy. It is related to the idea of power. Imagine an Omnipotent Being. An Omnipotent Being does not fear and does not need anything; thus It cannot hate nor hurt anyone. The only thing It can do is to give what It has. It *must* build and create, love and protect. Those who reach this point, the genuinely moral individuals, develop the *vector ego*. They have the courage to give. They do not need restraints: they are *autonomous*.

Becoming is synonymous with moral development which proceeds from irresponsible anomy through the borrowed responsibility of *heteronomy* toward the shared responsibility of *socionomy*. The next and the highest level of becoming is the individual's own responsibility: *autonomy*.

Autonomy means rules and commandments imposed from within. It implies a total and unreserved responsibility for whatever is going on. It is the moral obligation to fellow-man—to all men, women, and children. It is the ever-present readiness to be of help to those in need.

The ancient Persian religion of Zarathustra did not use punishment and reward as moral devices. It appealed to the innermost feeling of *responsibility*. According to this religion, the world is divided between the forces of light, symbolized by Ormuzd, the lofty God of Light, and Ahriman, the evil God of Darkness. The struggle between right and wrong, justice and evil, love and hate goes on in every human heart. Good deeds support Ormuzd, evil deeds help Ahriman.

Whose victory do you, the individual, want to bring? It is up to every human being to take sides in this struggle and every single individual is responsible for its outcome. Every human being is free to choose between love and hate. There is no reward or punishment, but only moral responsibility. It is the moral obligation to serve the God of Light and to give oneself to this task, even when no one else joins them.

Jeremiah condemned his sinful compatriots. The ancient Egyptian King Akhnaton, introduced a monotheistic faith in a single god, Aton, in opposition to the powerful pagan priests. Christ proclaimed love and charity, in opposition to the materialistic and oppressive Roman Empire. Johann Huss was burned alive when he called for a revival of Christ's moral principles. Martin Luther fought against papal corruption. Loving parents are not emotionally impoverished, and the more love they give the more love they have.

The more energy one uses, the more access he gains to the deeper layers of his psyche. Consider a gold mine; those who trample on the surface picking the exposed gold pieces do not save their gold resources, but those who dig deep gain access to real treasures.

Heteronomous individuals who obey orders from without use as much energy as is required of them. More energy is used by socionomous individuals who take an active part in the group decision-making process. But maximum energy is revealed by autonomous individuals who are free to use all their energies at will.

In economic life slaves are the least efficient workers; hired labor is more efficient, and free enterprise is the most efficient. No one works as hard and as productively as the men and women who work on their own.

Free spirits can produce many times more than mental slaves. People who have the courage to be themselves, who are free to live the way they want and set their own goals, gain access to their hidden energy sources.

People who yield to every temptation, unable to control themselves, are not free. They may become slaves to alcoholism, drugs, and violent behavior. They are at the mercy of their momentary impulses, pushed around by their own weakness.

Freedom means the freedom to make one's own decisions. Freedom means the power to control one's behavior, to set goals in life, and vigorously pursue them. Freedom to think and to develop new ideas and to choose one's way in life must not be confused with regression to infantile modes of behavior. One cannot reverse developmental process, and whoever tries to turn a tree into a sapling will ruin the tree; immature men and women do not turn into children but become disturbed, maladjusted adults.

Genuine freedom is attained through autonomy of the human mind. People capable of giving orders to themselves and of exercising full control over their cravings and desires, capable of reasoning and deciding, are free human beings.

6

Personality Integration

The Criteria

Every human being is a conglomeration of diverse and often conflicting drives, impulses, needs, feelings, and thoughts. Human nature resembles a piano with its numerous keys, any combination of which can play various melodies in different keys. Apparently not all pianos are well tuned, and not all personalities are well integrated.

But why integrate? Integration for what? What is the integrating goal? What are the criteria? Is it the pleasure versus pain continuum? Or success versus failure? Or tension versus relief? Or health versus disease (Carson, 1989)?

Certainly pleasure is pleasurable and pain is painful. But pleasure can be destructive and pain constructive. Consider the pleasure people derive from alcohol and drug abuse. Pain, on the other hand, serves usually as an alarm signal. Pain points to a disease or a deficiency that needs immediate intervention, and diseases that are not associated with pain can go on unnoticed and cause irreparable harm.

Is it, then, the success versus failure continuum? People usually prefer success, but is it always so? One's success is not necessarily a one-to-one result of one's intelligence, tenacity, and other virtues. A lot depends on unpredictable natural and/or human forces such as earthquakes, volcanoes, hurricanes, floods, wars, revolutions, and riots. Not everyone who succeeds in his attempts is a well-integrated person, and not everyone who loses money on Wallstreet or is mugged, hit by a car, or killed in war is a disorganized, poorly integrated individual.

Several scientists assumed that relief from tension represents the ideal state. Similar ideas were conveyed by Cannon's (1932) homeostasis, Freud's (1933) constancy principle, and Goldstein's (1939) principle of equilibrium. Pleasure, however, is not identical with relief from tension, and no organism ever attains a state of perfect equilibrium.

Consider sexual behavior. Orgasm brings relief, but sexual foreplay and sexual intercourse are states of intense and tense pleasure. Consider intake of food; eating a good meal brings relief from hunger, but does not bring a peaceful state of relief to the digestive system.

It seems that the health versus disease continuum offers the most sensible solution to the problem of personality integration.

MENTAL HEALTH

Any disease is a state of disorganization, disturbance, and disorder; health is a state of orderly functioning. Moreover, the concepts of health and disease are closely related to the fundamental issue of every human life, namely, life itself, and the degree of health is commensurable to the chances for survival. A healthy person has a better chance for satisfying his or her needs and survival is the arch need. Good physical health is a highly relevant ingredient in one's power, defined earlier in this book as the ability to satisfy needs.

A sick person has less power and therefore less chance for survival. The severity of a disease is measured by its distance from death. Accordingly, diseases can be graded starting with the mild one that does not jeopardize one's life through the severe ones, until the zero point of power, death (Kaplan and Camacho, 1983).

A similar reasoning could be applied to the concept of mental health. In contradistinction to physical health, the decline of mental health does not lead to death. However, severely disturbed individuals are unable to live unless someone takes care of them. Mildly disturbed individuals may not be able to adequately use their mental resources, and the severely disturbed ones may not be able to function at all. Adjustment to life is therefore the obvious criterion of mental health, for survival is the intrinsic and ultimate goal of all living organisms.

Survival is the name of the built-in purpose of life, and the concepts of personality integration, mental health, and so on cannot be discussed outside the context of life. Corpses are neither healthy nor sick, and death is neither normal nor abnormal. The behavior of living people can be life protecting or life damaging, healthy or morbid, adjustive or maladjustive. Personality can be integrated and survival directed, or disorganized and self-defeating (Hartman and Blankenstein, 1986).

The concept of mental health can be presented at least in two different ways, either as set of theoretical constructs or in observational terms. One may apply Freud's or modified Freudian constructs to present mental health as a sort of balance between the three parts of the mental apparatus: the id, ego, and superego. Consideration of dynamics, topography, and personality structure offers the proper framework for a Freudian concept of a well-adjusted and healthy person. Needless to say, such a person does not exist. The reasonably adjusted and more or less mentally healthy person may have his or her ups and downs and periods of crisis, but somehow manages to bounce back and restore the balance in the three areas of dynamics, topography, and structure.

The balance in dynamics implies a balance of cathexes between the Ares–destrudo and Eros–libido. The aretic–destructive cathexes must be balanced in a manner that provides adequate protection against one's enemies. A well-adjusted individual does not hate the entire world and is not motivated by an all-out paranoia, but is ready to fight those who threaten his survival and well-being. Object hypercathexis of destrudo directed against innocent people or hypocathexis of destrudo and denial of external threats are signs of mental disbalance and poor mental health.

The same reasoning applies to the intracathetic balance of destrudo. Hypercathexis of self-directed destrudo leads to self-defeating behavior and eventually to suicide.

The balance of libido cathexes seems to be of particular significance in psychopathology, for a reasonable balance of interindividual and intraindividual libido cathexes is usually indicative of good mental health. In well-adjusted individuals a considerable part of libido is self-invested; they take care of their own needs, avoid unnecessary risks, and act in a manner that protects their life and well-being. They are, however, capable of investing a considerable part of their libido in other people. They are reasonably selfish and reasonably unselfish; they love themselves and love others, too. The distribution of energy between the self-directed and object-directed cathexes fluctuates, but it never goes to extreme neglect of themselves nor to an extreme neglect of other

people. The balance of libido and destrudo in their relationship to oneself and to others is the most significant element
of personality integration.

The interactional classification of mental disorders (Krauss
and Krauss, 1977) is linked to the distribution of libido inter- and
intraindividual cathexes. I have suggested the division of all
psychogenic mental disorders into a *hyperinstrumental–narcissistic*
type whose libido is object-hypocathected and self-hypercathected;
this type corresponds to the traditional category of sociopaths
or psychopaths. The second type are the *hypervectorials* whose
libido is object-hypercathected and self-hypocathected, which
includes schizophrenia and the schizoid-type disorders. The
third type, the *dysmutuals* shift from one extreme to another;
hysterics and manic depressives belong to this type.

The dynamic theory provides the main criterion for personality integration and mental health and the concept of
mental health is synonymous with balance of inter- and intraindividual cathexes of libido. As it was explained in the
previous chapters, there are no developmental phases in destrudo, and pathology is indicated by lack of self-control and
impulsive aretic acting out or by an excessive self-control or
by projection of one's own hostility on others. Apparently,
aretic behavior or lack of it cannot serve as the sole criterion
of mental health. Observational criteria of mental health are
described as follows.

OBSERVATIONAL CRITERIA OF MENTAL HEALTH

The first observational criteria of mental health is the
relationship between one's potentialities and achievements.
The inability to actualize one's mental and physical potential
is one of the outstanding signs of mental disorder. All other
factors being equal, the greater the discrepancy between

promise and fulfillment, the more severe is the disorder (Matarazzo, 1978).

There are, however, cases of gifted individuals who function well in their professional lives as scholars, scientists, and creative artists, while unable to act in a balanced and rational manner in their personal lives and interindividual relations. Apparently, their poorly integrated personality structure permits adequate functioning in the conflict-free ego spheres but it fails in conflict-laden areas.

The second criterion of mental health is emotional balance. The reactions of healthy individuals are typically in accordance with the nature and magnitude of stimuli. Normally we react with pleasure and joy to situations that enhance our well-being. Happiness is generally attained when one's wishes come true, while grief is the reaction to failure or loss.

Normal emotional reaction is proportionate to the stimulus. Let us consider the case of a man who has lost money. Assuming that he is emotionally well-balanced, his reaction will be appropriate to the fact of loss and proportionate to its magnitude and to the ensuing financial hardship. The more money lost, the greater the degree of upset; if the loss is only a small fraction of his possessions, his worry will be mild and of short duration. A well-balanced individual will do whatever is possible to regain the loss and to prevent the recurrence of losses in the future. A rational, balanced, and mentally healthy individual reacts with disappointment to failure, his reaction is proportionate to the damage incurred, and his actions lead to reduction or alleviation of past troubles and prevention of future ones. In short, normal emotional behavior is appropriate, proportionate, and adjustive.

Disturbed individuals tend to persist in mourning and perpetuating their depressed or aggressive moods instead of compensating for past losses and preventing future misfortunes. Because their emotional balance cannot be easily restored, the depressed or agitated anxiety states are likely to occur again and again. The failure in coping with hardships often leads to increasing irritability, each new frustration adding to the difficulty in restoring emotional balance. It becomes apparent that mental disorder is a dynamic process with a distinct tendency toward deterioration (Millon, Green, and Meagher, 1982).

Emotional balance implies the ability to control one's emotions. As above explained, the newborn child's behavior is anomous. The behavior is a series of impulsive actions and instant reactions to stimuli, following the lust for life principle.

Emotionally disturbed individuals may react instantly to an annoying stimulus without considering potential dangers. They may perpetuate their mood, unable to control them. Rational behavior is distinguished by self-discipline and the ability to control overt expression of one's emotions.

The third criterion of mental health is related to the validity of cognitive functions. An erroneous perception, an oversight of danger, an inability to distinguish fantasy from reality seriously jeopardize one's existence. A realistic perception of what is going on in the outer world and in one's own life increases one's chances for survival and helps in optional adjustment.

In most mental disorders, the perception of the outer world is disturbed, but not as a result of some malfunction of the sensory organs as is the case in sight or hearing impairments. Nor is the reduced ability to perceive, compare, and reason a function of mental deficiency as is true of retarded individuals. The mental apparatus is, in most cases of mental disorder, fully or partly preserved, but it seems that the mentally disturbed individual is unable to properly utilize his mental capacities because of a malfunction in the realm of feelings.

The more one is disturbed, the poorer is his contact with reality. Everyone makes an occasional perceptual error, but as a rule we are accurate and capable of correcting our errors. In mentally disturbed individuals, this ability is impaired or nonexistent (Wolman, 1978).

The situation can become quite serious when the picture of the outer world is distorted. An individual who consistently misconstrues or misinterprets what he perceives is said to be *delusional*. For example, when a mentally disturbed individual flees a policeman who simply wants to check his driver's license, in fear that the policeman will arrest him for a non-committed crime, or when he ascribes hostile feelings to his friends who are loyal and trustworthy, his reality testing is practically nonexistent. Whereas delusions are distorted perceptions, hallucinations are creations out of nothingness. Hallucination is perception without external stimulation, such as seeing ghosts and hearing voices. A hallucinating patient is unable to distinguish his inner fears, wishes, and dreams from the outer world. His ability in reality testing is lost.

The fourth criterion is social adjustment. Men live in societies. They interact with one another in cooperation and competition, love and hate, peace and war. The term "social life" denotes both the friendly or cooperative and the hostile or competitive aspects of human interaction.

There are no ideal societies. Every social group has its share of the constructive life-preserving and cooperative factors, as well as the disruptive, destructive, and antisocial forces. When the forces of hate prevail, however, life and society perish. No society can afford a free display of hostile and disruptive forces. If these forces are innate in men, they must be checked; if they are learned patterns of behavior, they must be unlearned at least to a point where they do not threaten the survival of men. There is a great diversity in the prohibitive actions of social groups; some limit their "thou shalt not kill" restraint to the members of their own group only.

One of the criteria of mental health is, as stated above, the ability to cooperate with others. Mentally healthy individuals are capable of living on friendly terms with other members of their group. They are capable of cooperation and are willing to enter into social relations based on mutual respect, agreement, and responsibility. Normal adults accept and make commitments that they can honor. They may disagree with associates and understand why others may disagree with them. They may occasionally feel hostile, but their actions are generally kept under control. They may, however, fight in self-defense in a manner approved by their cultural group.

Elsewhere in this volume three types of social interactions have been introduced, namely, instrumental, mutual, and vectorial. A well-integrated individual can act in all three levels. He or she is instrumental in breadwinning behavior, mutual in relationships with close friends, marriage, and sex, and vectorial in regard to children and those who need help, and in pursuit of ideas.

A realistic perception of the world is probably the most important criterion of mental health. An individual who does not see things the way they are and is plagued by delusions and/or hallucinations is definitely severely maladjusted.

The same applies to the way one sees oneself. Individuals who do not perceive themselves correctly may run into tremendous difficulties in life. If they overestimate their abilities, they may do things that will inevitably bring frustration and defeat. If they underestimate their own abilities, they may be afraid to do useful things that present no threat and they will therefore be doomed to remain underachievers.

Awareness of oneself does not imply an unconditional acceptance of one's faults and shortcomings. Awareness of oneself is the awareness of the fact that here are the cards that one got from heredity and experience and one must play his cards the best he can.

A person may realize that if he or she tends to be belligerent, the belligerence can be used for an active life, such as, for instance, conquering disease or misery and not necessarily for fighting people. One may neutralize some of his energies or sublimate some of them. One does not necessarily accept all the aspects of his or her own personality nor must one experiment with all possibilities. One must make selective decisions between the various possibilities and choose his or her way in life. Living in accordance with what one believes is a prerequisite of self-esteem, but the choices one must make are rarely self-evident and seldom easy ones.

POWER AND SELF-ESTEEM

The fundamental, innate, *basic* needs are oxygen, water, food, rest, shelter, sex, and so on. The *acquired* needs are to be accepted, protected, loved, respected, and so on.

Were human beings immortal, they would have no needs whatsoever. Were human beings mortal but omnipotent, they would have the basic needs only. Their weakness makes them totally dependent on others during their infancy and less dependent in adulthood. The more power they have, the less they depend on others.

Self-esteem depends on awareness of one's power. An individual who perceives himself as physically healthy, attractive, intelligent, influential, or outstanding in any way has the feeling of power defined as the ability to satisfy needs. If he likes to ski and is a good skier, he has the feeling of "ski-power." If he is materialistic and has a good income or substantial possessions, he has the feeling of "money-power."

This or any other power is tantamount to a high degree of self-esteem. Since no human being is omnipotent, lack of acceptance and support from without makes one feel weak and therefore lowers his or her self-esteem. Self-esteem may or may not correspond to reality and it may be a product of a rational or irrational estimate of one's own power and the power and loyalty of one's allies.

Little children are not capable of precise perception or of a sober judgment. When a little boy draws a picture of a dog, he may not notice that his dog has too little or too many legs. He depends on daddy or mommy; if they criticize his work, they undermine his self-confidence and self-esteem; if they praise, they encourage and enhance his self-confidence and self-esteem. Parental opinion is the prime source of either self-assuredness or of inferiority feelings.

As the child grows older, the interaction with peers and adults affects the child's self-confidence and self-esteem. A child who was encouraged at home has a better chance to win the approval of the peer group and, whenever necessary, to stand up to peer rejection. A child who comes to the nursery school, kindergarten, or grammar school with a feeling of inferiority may avoid social contacts and is likely to be rejected. As years go by the feeling of one's own worthlessness makes one more and more dependent on what other people think of him or her, and the more one needs approval, the slimmer are the chances to obtain it.

People whose self-confidence was built-up in childhood have more courage and depend less on others. One's own abilities, efforts, and achievements gradually count more than whatever other people's opinions may be. Self-respecting and self-confident men and women depend less on what others think of them than what they think of themselves. Well-adjusted people are aware of the fact that not everyone is going to like them, and therefore they act in accordance with what *they themselves* think is right. The dependence on one's own judgment is a crucial ingredient in personality integration and mental health, provided it is based on a realistic estimate of one's own potentialities and environmental opportunities.

Courage to be oneself is a highly important element of self-esteem. Courage implies faith in oneself and it indicates self-confidence and self-reliance. It represents the belief that one has the power to stand up and be counted.

Everyone's life has ups and downs, but brave men and women act courageously in victory and defeat, in success and failure. True courage is related to a realistic estimate of one's own power and the power of the threatening forces. Brave men and women take necessary precautions and use good judgment whenever they have to face a challenge and they make responsible decisions.

ACHIEVING

One of the most realistic aspects of life is economic life. Economic means are a realistic sign of power, realistic in the sense that those who have can do more things that those who do not have. Food, shelter, clothing, and entertainment are bought with money, and the more money one has, the easier it is for a person to satisfy his needs and the needs of people who depend on him. Economic power is one of the most tangible signs: Those who are rich have more power; those who are poor have less.

Self-esteem is the feeling of power; people who think highly of themselves in terms of power respect themselves, that is, they have a high degree of self-esteem. Certainly it is no one-to-one relationship, and there are a great many people who accomplished a lot in economic life and still suffer a lack of self-esteem. However, the feeling of economic achievement is likely to give one a good deal of the feeling of power. There is more to making money than to having it. Climbing mountains, overcoming obstacles, and forging ahead gives one a wonderful feeling of power. The road full of obstacles offers more challenges and, therefore, more opportunities for triumph. Reaching the greatest heights and doing what seems to be impossible is a great source of pride and joy.

There is an additional benefit in economic success. In our society money and economic success elicit a great deal of respect and improve one's social status. Social status is the position one has with regard to others as perceived by others. In our society, economic achievement and wealth are one of the most outstanding features that commands respect. The approval by others and esteem given by them reinforces one's self-esteem; in most cases people enjoy the approval of others because this reinforces in them additional feelings of power and success.

In addition to these tangible successes there are also more subtle and sublime ways by which people can attain the feeling of power. A scientist who makes great discoveries may derive a tremendous feeling of power; the same applies to a writer, a painter, or a composer. All these achievements, all these accomplishments give one the feeling of power and are a great source of pride and happiness.

Behind all these desires, strivings, and achievements lies the conscious or unconscious wish to overcome the fear of the inevitable. Men and women who have attained physical, political, economic, intellectual, or artistic power, who have children and take pride in them, consciously or unconsciously cherish the idea that if they cannot physically survive death, their children, their deeds, their works, their fortunes, their achievements, and creations will last forever.

FIELD-THEORETICAL CONSIDERATIONS

Human beings do not live in a vacuum and the content of their wishes and cravings is greatly influenced by their environment. It has been frequently observed that even the same person may act in different ways in different environments. Lewin (1951) and Sullivan (1953) went so far as to assume that it is impossible to assert one's personality outside his or her social environment. These field-theoretical hypotheses have some merit, although one should not go to the extreme. One is what one is, but how one uses his resources, abilities, and experiences greatly depends on interactional patterns.

The concept of interindividual cathexis might be applied at this point. The same child will behave in a totally different manner at home where he or she feels rejected than at grandmother's where they feel accepted. To be rejected means receiving no or very little supply of libido cathexes and probably plenty of destrudo cathexes in the form of criticism, scolding, and punishments. Parental rejection evokes in the child interindividual destrudo cathexes ("I hate my parents") and probably also intraindividual destrudo cathexes ("I must not deserve love; I hate myself"). These feelings must lead to temporary or lasting changes in child's personality. The changes may be suspended, pushed aside, or repressed in the child's interaction with his affectionate grandmother. The grandmother "gives the child her love," that is, she cathects some of her libido into the child. The child's personality, as it were, becomes enriched by the gift of love.

Thus the most plausible interpretation is that the external factor somehow transmits part of its energetic load into the peripheral endings of a centripetal nerve, that is, cathects this nerve ending and changes it.

Apparently, certain people and certain situations elicit different reactions in the same people. As mentioned at the beginning of this chapter the human mind resembles a piano with a great many keys. It is, indeed, the same instrument, but it can give different melodies in different keys. The basic elements of one's personality are there, but some of them come to the fore in different situations.

There are no clear-cut distinctions between the various ethnic, racial, or religious groups. There are breathtaking differences within each group, and there are a great many bright and dull, fair and unfair, friendly and hostile Czechs, Irish, Jewish, black, Chinese, and Mexican people. There is no reason to assume that *all* Italians or *all* Germans or *all* Russians are alike, but living together in physical proximity, sharing the same social and economic institutions, and being exposed to the same cultural, religious, and political ideas must influence people's feelings, thoughts, and actions. The environmental influences cannot reach the genetically determined parts of personality, and the id part of human nature with its basic lust for life and aretic and erotic drives probably do not change. The way people endeavor to satisfy their basic needs and how they feel about themselves and others, however, greatly depends on environmental influences, starting with parents, teachers, and sociocultural trends.

People's egos, superegos, we-egos, and vector-egos are considerably influenced by their life experiences and the physical, sociocultural, economic, and political climate of their times. One must not conclude that all Frenchmen act in a certain way and all Saudis in another, but one should look for common behavioral patterns that develop within a given society at a given time. In other words, the sociopsychological field of most Americans is certainly different from the sociopsychological field of most people in the Soviet Union,

China, Switzerland, or Chile, although all people everywhere in the world have certain fundamental common needs and share certain personality elements common to the entire human race (Adler, 1973).

THE MEANING OF LIFE

There are three main turning points in human life; the first one is birth. No one has ever asked to be born and no one influences the start of his or her life. Birth, the fundamental fact of one's life, is totally beyond one's control. Also, the last, terminal moment of one's life does not offer much choice either. Old age, sickness, or accidents put an end to every human life, be that of a sage or a fool, a king or a pauper.

Between these two great events, which are determined without one's approval, there is one decision that one can make if he or she understands its importance and urgency: It is the decision of how to live and with whom to live—the third crucial point on which every individual *can* exercise considerable influence. Children's lives are controlled and regulated by parents or parental substitutes but adults can make their choice of occupation, of place of residence, and the way they intend to live. They must be aware of the causal relationship: Whatever they do will produce certain effects.

The decision-making process should start with a realistic appraisal of what life is about. The fact is that life as such has no intrinsic meaning. Human life is a biological process, just as the life of any other organism. Moreover, people are born before they are ready to live and they may die just when they begin to live.

No one lives in a vacuum and no one has all the options. Heredity and environment offer different opportunities and set different limits for each individual. Life itself is the common denominator of all the options.

Life is an unrepeatable chance and an unsolicited gift. To be alive is a prerequisite to whatever joy, pleasure, satisfaction, and happiness one can experience. To miss the opportunity of using one's options is a crime and a punishment. It is a crime not to walk when one has legs; it is a crime not to sing, not to smile, not to give, not to enjoy, and the crime brings a most severe punishment—the punishment of futility, of meaningless vegetation and wasted life.

No one can achieve more than he can achieve considering his or her *innate* potentialities, such as health, intelligence, and so on, and the external opportunities, such as home background, education, peers, economic factors, and the entire fabric of economic, political, and cultural relations of his time. Considering the totality of factors, no one can be an overachiever.

Unfortunately, a great many people realize but a fraction of their potentialities and are underachievers. An underachiever is one who accomplishes much *less* than his capabilities and circumstances permit.

Human life is a sheer coincidence: a certain sperm cell meets with an egg cell. There is no purpose in life nor is there any purpose in death. Some tissues fade just away, some muscles get tired of working, some hearts stop beating, or some bullets interrupt the process of life.

The truth is simple and obvious: There is no self-evident purpose to human life.

All human beings know that life is a gift that can be revoked at any time. In fact, life is the only thing we have.

Human beings have nothing else but their years of life. And no matter what we think about, no matter what we do, love, hate, philosophize, defend, reject, there is only one thing: life itself.

References

Adler, A. *The practice and theory of individual psychology.* London: Routledge & Kegan Paul, 1929.

Adler, L.L. *Aggression: A social learning analysis.* Englewood Cliffs: NJ: Prentice-Hall, 1973.

Bandura, A. *Aggression: A social learning analysis.* Englewood Cliffs, NJ: Prentice-Hall, 1973.

Bassin, F.W. *The problem of the unconscious.* (Russian). Moscow: Medical Publishing, 1968.

Beauvoir, S. de. *The second sex.* New York: Knopf, 1953.

Bellak, L., and Fielding, C. Diagnosing schizophrenia. In B.B. Wolman (Ed.), *Clinical diagnosis of mental disorders: A handbook*, pp. 757–774. New York: Plenum, 1978.

Bevan, W., Daves, W.F., and Levy, G. W. The relation of castration, androgen therapy and pre-test fighting experience to competitive aggression in male C57BL/10 mice. *Animal Behavior,* 1960, *8,* 6–12.

Bohm, D. *Causality and chance in modern physics.* New York: Harper & Row, 1957.

Brehm, J.W., and Self, E.A. The intensity of motivation. In M.R. Rosenzweig and L.W. Porter (Eds.), *Annual review of psychology,* vol. 40, pp. 109–131. Palo Alto, Calif.: Annual Reviews, 1989.

Bridgman, P.W. *The logic of modern physics.* New York: Macmillan, 1927.

Bridgman, P.W. *The nature of physical theory.* Princeton: Princeton University Press, 1936.

Burlingham, D., and Freud, A. *Young children in wartime.* London: Allen and Unwin, 1942.

Bykov, K. *The cerebral cortex and the inner organs.* New York: Chemical Publishers, 1957.

Cannon, W.B. *Bodily changes in pain, hunger, fear and rage.* New York: Appleton-Century, 1932.

Carmichael, L. The onset and early development of behavior. In L. Carmichael (Ed.), *Manual of child psychology.* New York: Wiley, 1954.

Carson, R. Personality. In M.R. Rosenzwieg and L.W. Porter (Eds.), *Annual review of psychology,* vol. 40, pp. 227–248. Palo Alto, Calif.: Annual Reviews, 1989.

Caudill, W. *The psychiatric hospital as a small society.* Cambridge, MA: Harvard University Press, 1958.

Chari, C. T. K. Some generalized theories and models of PSI: A critical evaluation. In B.B. Wolman (Ed.), *Handbook of parapsychology.* Jefferson, NC: McFarland, 1986.

Chertok, L. Reinstatement of the concept of the unconscious in the Soviet Union. *American Journal of Psychiatry,* 1981, *138,* 575–583.

Cobb, S. *Foundations of neuropsychiatry.* Baltimore, Md.: Williams and Wilkins, 1958.

Comte, A. *Cours de philosophie positive.* Paris: Baillere, 1864.

Descartes, R. *Philosohical works.* 2 vols. Cambridge: Cambridge University Press, 1931.

Deutsch, F. (Ed.). *On the mysterious lead from the mind to the body.* New York: International Universities Press, 1959.

Eccles, J., *The nerophysiological basis of mind.* New York: McGraw-Hill, 1953.

Einstein, A. *The World as I see it.* New York: Friede, 1934.

Einstein, A. Reply to criticism. In P.A. Schilpp (Ed.), *Albert Einstein: philosopher-scientist,* vol. 2. New York: Harper & Row, 1959.

Eissler, K. R. *Thanassa.* New York: International Universities Press, 1955.

Erikson, E. *Childhood and society.* New York: Norton, 1963.

Feigl, H. Principles and problems of theory construction in psychology. In W. Dennis (Ed.), *Current trends in psychological theory.* Pittsburgh, PA: University of Pittsburgh Press, 1951.

Filskov, S. B., and Boll, T. J. (Eds.). *Handbook of clinical neuropsychology.* New York: Wiley, 1981.

Firsoff, V. A. *Life, mind and galaxies.* Edinburgh: Oliver and Boyd, 1967.

Fiss, H. Current dream research: A psychobiological perspective. In B.B. Wolman (Ed.), *Handbook of dreams,* pp. 20–74. New York: Van Nostrand Reinhold, 1979.

Freud, S. *Beyond the pleasure principle* (1920). New York: Liveright, 1950.

Freud, S. *New introductory lectures on psychoanalysis.* New York: Norton, 1933.

Freud, S. *An outline of psychoanalysis* (1938). New York: Norton, 1949.

Fromm, E. *Escape from freedom.* New York: Farrar and Rinehart, 1941.

Fuller, J. L., and Simmel, E. *Behavior genetics: Principles and applications.* Hillsdale, NJ: Erlbaum, 1983.

Garmezy, N. Stimulus differentiation by schizophrenic and normal subjects under conditions of reward and punishment. *Journal of Personality,* 1952, *20,* 253–276.

Gesell, A. Maturation and the patterning of behavior. In C. Murchison (Ed.), *Handbook of child psychology.* Worcester, MA: Clark University Press, 1928.

Gilgen, A. R. (Ed.). *Contemporary scientific psychology.* New York: Academic Press, 1970.

Goldstein, K. *The organism.* New York: American Book, 1939.

Guthrie, E. R. *The psychology of learning.* New York: Harper & Row, 1935.

Hamburg, D. A., and Trudeau, M. (Eds.). *Behavioral aspects of aggression.* New York: Liss, 1981.

Harmony, T. *Functional neuroscience.* Hillsdale, NJ: Earlbaum, 1984.

Hartman, L. M., and Blankstein, K. R. (Eds.). *Perception of self in emotional disorder and psychotherapy.* New York: Plenum, 1986.

Hegel, G. W. F. *Phenomenologie des Geistes.* Berlin: Duncker and Humbolt, 1841.

Horney, K. *New ways in psychoanalysis.* New York: Norton, 1939.

Hull, C. L. The problem of intervening variables in motor behavior theory. *Psychological Review,* 1943, *50,* 273–291.

Irani, K. D., Conceptual changes in the problem of mind–body relations. In R.W. Riebey (Ed.), *Body and mind.* New York: Academic Press, 1980.

Jeans, J. *Physics and philosophy.* Ann Arbor: University of Michigan Press, 1958.

Kahana, B. Social behavior and aging. In B.B. Wolman (Ed.), *Handbook of developmental psychology*, pp. 871–889. Englewood Cliffs, NJ: Prentice Hall, 1982.

Kant, I. *Critique of pure reason*, 2nd ed. (Trans. N. Kemp Smith) London: Macmillan, 1929.

Kaplan, G. A., and Camacho, T. Perceived health and mortality: A nine year follow-up of the human population laboratory cohort. *American Journal of Epidemiology*, 1983, *117*, 292–304.

Keith, C. R. (Ed.) *The aggressive adolescent*. New York: Free Press, 1984.

Krauss, H. H., and Krauss, B. J. Nosology: Wolman's system. In B.B. Wolman (Ed.), *International encyclopedia of psychiatry, psychology, psychoanalysis and neurology*, vol. 8, pp. 86–88. New York: Van Nostrand/Aesculapius, 1977.

LaBerge, S. *Awake in your dreams: The new world of lucid dreaming*. New York: Simon & Schuster, 1984.

Lewin, K. *Principles of topological psychology*. New York: McGraw-Hill, 1936.

Lewin, K. *The conceptual representation and the measurement of psychological forces*. University of Iowa: *Contributions to Psychological Theory*, 1938, *1*(4).

Lewin, K. *Field theory in social science*. New York: Harper & Row, 1951.

Locke, J. *An essay concerning human understanding*. Oxford: Oxford University Press, 1894.

Lorenz, K. *On aggression*. New York: Harcourt Brace Jovanovich 1966.

Maccoby, E. E. Socialization and developmental change. *Child Development*, 1984, *55*, 317–328.

Mach, E. *History and root of the principle of the conservation of energy* (1872). La Salle, IL: Open Court, 1911.

Mach, E. *The science of mechanics*. Chicago: Open Court, 1960.

Maslow, A. *Toward a psychology of being*. New York: Van Nostrand Reinhold, 1968.

Matarazzo, J. D. The interview: Its reliability and validity in psychiatric diagnosis. In B.B. Wolman (Ed.), *Clinical diagnosis of mental disorders: A handbook*. New York: Plenum, 1978.

Mead, M. *Male and female*. New York: Morrow, 1950.

Mednick, S. A., and Christiansen, K. O. (Eds.). *Biosocial bases of criminality*. New York: Gardner, 1980.

Millon, T., Green, C., and Meagher, R. (Eds.). *Handbook of clinical health psychology*. New York: Plenum, 1982.

Montagu, M. F. A. *Prenatal influences*. Springfield, IL: Thomas, 1962.

Murphy, G. *Personality*. New York: Harper & Row, 1947.

Nagel, E. *The structure of science*. New York: Harcourt Brace, 1961.

Northrop, F. S. C. Einstein's conception of science. In P.A. Schilpp (Ed.), *Albert Einstein: Philosopher-scientist*. New York: Harper & Row, 1959.

Noyes, A. P., and Kolb, L. C. *Modern clinical psychiatry*, 5th ed. Philadelphia: Saunders, 1959.

Oparin, A. I. *The origins of life on earth*. New York: Academic Press, 1957.

Pavlov, I. P. *Lectures on conditioned reflexes*. New York: Liveright, 1928.

Poincaré, H. *La science et l'hypothese*. Paris: Flammarion, 1902.

Popper, K. L. *The logic of scientific discovery*. New York: Basic Books, 1961.

Pribram, K. H., and Gill, M. *Freud's project reassessed*. New York: Basic Books, 1966.

Razran, G. Soviet psychology since 1950. *Science*, 1957, *126*, 1100–1107.

Rowan-Robinson, M. *Cosmology*. New York: Oxford University Press, 1981.

Rychlak, J. F. The nature and challenge of teleological psychological theory. *Annals of Theoretical Discovery*, 1984, *2*, 115–150.

Schopenhauer, A. *The world as will and idea*. New York: Scribner, 1923.

Sheffield, F. D., and Roby, T. B. Reward value of nonnutritive sweet tastes. *Journal of Comparative and Physiological Psychology*, 1950, *43*, 471–481.

Stanton, A. H., and Schwartz, M. S. *The mental hospital: A study of institutional participation in psychiatric illness and treatment*. New York: Basic Books, 1951.

Stechler, G., and Halton, A. Prenatal influences on human development. In B.B. Wolman (Ed.), *Handbook of developmental psychology*, pp. 175–189. Englewood Cliffs, NJ: Prentice-Hall, 1982.

Sullivan, G. S. *Interpersonal theory of psychiatry*. New York: Norton, 1953.

Tschakhotine, S. Reactions conditionnés par micropuncture ultraviolette dans le comportement d'une cellule isolée. *Archives d'Institute Prophylactique*, 1938, *10*, 113–119.

Valzelli, L. *Psychobiology of aggression and violence*. New York: Rowen, 1981.

Vandenberg, S. G., and Vogler, G. P. Genetic determinants of intelligence. In B.B. Wolman (Ed.), *Handbook of intelligence*, pp. 3–57. New York: Wiley, 1985.

Williams, J. A. *Psychology of women.* New York: Norton, 1977.

Winder, C. L. Some psychological studies of schizophrenics. In Jackson, D. D. (Ed.), *The etiology of schizophrenia.* New York: Basic Books, 1960.

Wolman, B. B. The Antigone principle. *American Imago,* 1965, *22,* 186–201.

Wolman, B. B. *Vectoriasis Praecox or the Group of Schizophrenias.* Springfield, IL: Charles C. Thomas, 1966.

Wolman, B. B. *Psychoanalytic techniques.* New York: Basic Books, 1967.

Wolman, B. B. (Ed.), *Historical roots of contemporary psychology.* New York: Harper & Row, 1968.

Wolman, B. B. Concerning psychology and the philosophy of science. In B.B. Wolman (Ed.), *Handbook of general psychology.* Englewood Cliffs, NJ: Prentice-Hall, 1973.

Wolman, B. B. *Children without childhood.* New York: Grune and Stratton, 1970.

Wolman, B. B. (Ed.). *Clinical diagnosis of mental disorders: A handbook.* New York: Plenum, 1978.

Wolman, B. B. *Contemporary theories and systems in psychology.* New York: Plenum, 1981.

Wolman, B. B. (Ed.). *Handbook of developmental psychology.* Englewood Cliffs, NJ: Prentice-Hall, 1982.

Wolman, B. B. *The logic of science in psychoanalysis.* New York: Columbia University Press, 1984.

Wolman, B. B. (Ed.), *Handbook of intelligence: Theories, measurements, and applications.* New York: Wiley Interscience, 1985.

Wolman, B. B. Monistic transitionism. In B.B. Wolman (Ed.), *Handbook of parapsychology.* Jefferson, NC: McFarland, 1986.

Wolman, B. B. *Sociopathic personality.* New York: Brunner-Mazel, 1987.

Wolman, B. B. *Psychosomatic disorders.* New York: Plenum, 1988.

Wolman, B. B., and Money, J. (Eds.). *Handbook of human sexuality.* Englewood Cliffs, NJ: Prentice-Hall, 1980.

Wolman, B. B., and Nagel, E. (Eds.). *Scientific psychology.* New York: Basic Books, 1965.

Wolman, B. B., and Stricker, G. (Eds.). *Handbook of family and marital therapy.* New York: Plenum, 1983.

Wolman, B. B., and Stricker, G. (Eds.). *Depressive disorders*. New York: Wiley, 1990.

Ziferstein, I. Union of Soviet Socialist Republics: personality theory. In B.B. Wolman (Ed.), *International encyclopedia of psychiatry, psychology, psychoanalysis and neurology: Progress*, vol. 1, pp. 466–471. New York: Aesculapius, 1983.

Author Index

157

Subject Index